Psychosocial Interventions in Mental Health Nursing

Transforming Nursing Practice series

Transforming Nursing Practice is a series of books designed to help students meet the requirements of the NMC Standards and Essential Skills Clusters for degree programmes. Each book addresses a core topic, and together they cover the generic knowledge required for all fields of practice.

Core knowledge titles:

Series editor: Professor Shirley Bach, Head of the School of Health Sciences at the University of Brighton

Acute and Critical Care in Adult Nursing	ISBN 978 0 85725 842 7
Becoming a Registered Nurse: Making the Transition to Practice	ISBN 978 0 85725 931 8
Caring for Older People in Nursing	ISBN 978 1 44626 763 9
Communication and Interpersonal Skills in Nursing (2nd edn)	ISBN 978 0 85725 449 8
Contexts of Contemporary Nursing (2nd edn)	ISBN 978 1 84445 374 0
Dementia Care in Nursing	ISBN 978 0 85725 873 1
Getting into Nursing	ISBN 978 0 85725 895 3
Health Promotion and Public Health for Nursing Students (2nd edn)	ISBN 978 1 44627 503 0
Introduction to Medicines Management in Nursing	ISBN 978 1 84445 845 5
Law and Professional Issues in Nursing (3rd edn)	ISBN 978 1 44626 858 2
Leadership, Management and Team Working in Nursing	ISBN 978 0 85725 453 5
Learning Skills for Nursing Students	ISBN 978 1 84445 376 4
Medicines Management in Adult Nursing	ISBN 978 1 84445 842 4
Medicines Management in Children's Nursing	ISBN 978 1 84445 470 9
Nursing Adults with Long Term Conditions	ISBN 978 0 85725 441 2
Nursing and Collaborative Practice (2nd edn)	ISBN 978 1 84445 373 3
Nursing and Mental Health Care	ISBN 978 1 84445 467 9
Nursing in Partnership with Patients and Carers:	ISBN 978 0 85725 307 1
Passing Calculations Tests for Nursing Students (2nd edn)	ISBN 978 1 44625 642 8
Palliative and End of Life Care in Nursing	ISBN 978 1 44627 092 9
Patient and Carer Participation in Nursing	ISBN 978 0 85725 307 1
Patient Assessment and Care Planning in Nursing	ISBN 978 0 85725 858 8
Patient Safety and Managing Risk in Nursing	ISBN 978 1 44626 688 5
Psychology and Sociology in Nursing	ISBN 978 0 85725 836 6
Safeguarding Adults in Nursing Practice	ISBN 978 1 44625 638 1
Successful Practice Learning for Nursing Students (2nd edn)	ISBN 978 0 85725 315 6
Understanding Ethics for Nursing Students	ISBN 978 1 44627 126 1
Using Health Policy in Nursing	ISBN 978 1 44625 646 6
What is Nursing? Exploring Theory and Practice (3rd edn)	ISBN 978 0 85725 975 2

Personal and professional learning skills titles:

Series editors: Dr Mooi Standing, Independent Academic Consultant (UK and International) & Accredited NMC Reviewer and Professor Shirley Bach, Head of the School of Health Sciences at the University of Brighton

Clinical Judgement and Decision Making in for Nursing Students (2nd edn)	ISBN 978 1 44628 281 6
Critical Thinking and Writing for Nursing Students (2nd edn)	ISBN 978 1 44625 644 2
Evidence-based Practice in Nursing (2nd edn)	ISBN 978 1 44627 090 5
Information Skills for Nursing Students	ISBN 978 1 84445 381 8
Reflective Practice in Nursing (2nd edn)	ISBN 978 1 44627 085 1
Succeeding in Essays, Exams & OSCEs for Nursing Students	ISBN 978 0 85725 827 4
Succeeding in Literature Reviews and Research Project Plans for Nursing Students (2nd edn)	ISBN 978 1 44628 283 0
Successful Professional Portfolios for Nursing Students	ISBN 978 0 85725 457 3
Understanding Research for Nursing Students (2nd edn)	ISBN 978 1 44626 761 5

Mental health nursing titles:

Series editors: Sandra Walker, Senior Teaching Fellow in Mental Health in the Faculty of Health Sciences, University of Southampton and Professor Shirley Bach, Head of the School of Health Sciences at the University of Brighton

Assessment and Decision Making in Mental Health Nursing	ISBN 978 1 44626 820 9
Engagement and Therapeutic Communication in Mental Health Nursing	ISBN 978 1 44627 480 4
Medicines Management in Mental Health Nursing	ISBN 978 0 85725 049 0
Mental Health Law in Nursing	ISBN 978 0 85725 761 1
Physical Healthcare and Promotion in Mental Health Nursing	ISBN 978 1 44626 818 6
Psychosocial Interventions in Mental Health Nursing	ISBN 978 1 44627 508 5

You can find more information on each of these titles and our other learning resources at www.sagepub.co.uk. Many of these titles are also available in various e-book formats, please visit our website for more information.

Psychosocial Interventions in Mental Health Nursing

Edited by Sandra Walker

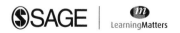

Los Angeles | London | New Delhi
Singapore | Washington DC

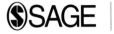

Learning Matters
An imprint of SAGE Publications Ltd
1 Oliver's Yard
55 City Road
London EC1Y 1SP

SAGE Publications Inc.
2455 Teller Road
Thousand Oaks, California 91320

SAGE Publications India Pvt Ltd
B 1/I 1 Mohan Cooperative Industrial Area
Mathura Road
New Delhi 110 044

SAGE Publications Asia-Pacific Pte Ltd
3 Church Street
#10-04 Samsung Hub
Singapore 049483

Editor: Alex Clabburn
Development editor: Caroline Sheldrick
Production controller: Chris Marke
Project management: Swales & Willis Ltd, Exeter, Devon
Marketing manager: Tamara Navaratnam
Cover design: Wendy Scott
Typeset by: C&M Digitals (P) Ltd, Chennai, India
Printed by: Henry Ling Limited at The Dorset Press, Dorchester, DT1 1HD

Introduction and editorial arrangement © Sandra Walker 2015
Chapter 1 © Wendy Turton
Chapter 2 © Simon Grist
Chapter 3 © Julie Roberts
Chapter 4 © Julie Roberts
Chapter 5 © Simon Grist, Peter Bullard and Janine Ward
Chapter 6 © Simon Grist
Chapter 7 © Kim Moore

First published 2015

Apart from any fair dealing for the purposes of research or private study, or criticism or review, as permitted under the Copyright, Designs and Patents Act, 1988, this publication may be reproduced, stored or transmitted in any form, or by any means, only with the prior permission in writing of the publishers, or in the case of reprographic reproduction, in accordance with the terms of licences issued by the Copyright Licensing Agency. Enquiries concerning reproduction outside those terms should be sent to the publishers.

Library of Congress Control Number: 2014947113

British Library Cataloguing in Publication data

A catalogue record for this book is available from the British Library

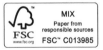

ISBN 978-1-4462-7507-8
ISBN 978-1-4462-7508-5 (pbk)

At SAGE we take sustainability seriously. Most of our products are printed in the UK using FSC papers and boards. When we print overseas we ensure sustainable papers are used as measured by the Egmont grading system. We undertake an annual audit to monitor our sustainability.

Contents

About the authors   vi
Foreword   viii
Acknowledgements   ix

Introduction   1

1   An introduction to psychosocial interventions   4
    Wendy Turton

2   Cognitive behavioural therapy   22
    Simon Grist

3   Dialectical behavioural therapy: an introduction   37
    Julie Roberts

4   Mindfulness for all in action   63
    Julie Roberts

5   Low intensity cognitive behavioural therapy interventions   81
    Simon Grist, Peter Bullard and Janine Ward

6   Why should I get fit? Physical activity as an intervention   107
    Simon Grist

7   Dual diagnosis   125
    Kim Moore

References   147
Index   157

About the authors

Peter Bullard

Peter Bullard is the Accredited Psychological Wellbeing Practitioner (PWP) Quality Lead for Isle of Wight Primary Care Mental Health service. He works with individuals suffering with anxiety and depression and delivers low intensity CBT interventions through different modalities. He graduated from Southampton University in 2010 and has worked on the course as a clinical educator since the same year. He has an MSc in Transcultural Mental Health and Psychological Therapies. Before working in mental health services he had a background in physical fitness, completing his degree in Health and Fitness management and working as an instructor and trainer in many different healthcare settings. He strongly believes in the value of combining therapeutic approaches with the application of improving wellbeing for individuals experiencing mental health problems.

Simon Grist

Simon Grist is a Lecturer in Mental Health and Programme Lead for the Improving Access to Psychological Therapies Psychological Wellbeing Practitioner programme at the University of Southampton. A qualified mental health nurse and CBT therapist, prior to working at the university he was a CMHT manager, working extensively in crisis and home treatment teams and in substance misuse services.

Kim Moore

Kim Moore (RMN, MSc Addictive Behaviour, PgCert Health Promotion and Approved Mental Health Practitioner) is currently a Lecturer in Mental Health with the Faculty of Health at Birmingham City University. Kim trained in Perth, Western Australia as a mental health nurse before moving to London in 1990. She has focused her career in working in substance misuse and mental health services, and in particular dual diagnosis. Kim has worked in a number of clinical and management positions during her career and in 1999 she helped design and establish the Haringey Dual Diagnosis Service. Kim worked as the service manager for dual diagnosis services in Haringey for seven years before taking on a nurse consultant role in Dual Diagnosis in Kent. Kim has been involved in developing dual diagnosis resources as a member of the National Nurse Consultants Group (PROGRESS) in partnership with the National Mental Health Development Unit. Kim remains involved in substance misuse and dual diagnosis education and practice.

Julie Roberts

Julie Roberts has experienced borderline personality disorder at first hand and has undertaken dialectical behavioural therapy and mindfulness training. Since completing she has been actively involved in teaching mindfulness and DBT skills in both in and outpatient settings, taught mindfulness at a local sixth form college and acts as an expert patient at Southampton University. In this role she has presented in conferences and taught groups of students, sits on the Expert by Experience and Lived Experience Groups and has participated in module design and revalidation.

Wendy Turton

Wendy Turton (RMN, MSc, BABCP Accred. Cognitive Therapist) is currently a Lecturer in Mental Health with the Faculty of Health Sciences at the University of Southampton and the Senior Psychological Therapist with a Mental Health Recovery Team in Portsmouth. Wendy trained in Leicestershire on an integrated Mental Health and Learning Disability nursing programme, choosing to focus her career on mental health and in recent years on severe and enduring mental health problems, in particular the experience of psychosis. In 2004 Wendy set up the Psychosocial Interventions for Psychosis Service (PSIPS) within South East Hampshire which she led for nine years. During this time Wendy was involved in clinical research exploring the efficacy of Person-Based Cognitive Therapy for Distressing Psychosis (Chadwick, 2006) and co-authored two award-winning short books on the experience of living with psychosis with MH service users; her ongoing research continues to focus on the lived experience of living with psychosis. Wendy also works with the CBT Programme Team at the University of Southampton.

Sandra Walker (editor)

Sandra Walker is a Senior Teaching Fellow in Mental Health at Southampton University where she is also a doctorate student researching the patient experience of mental health assessment in the Emergency Department. She is a qualified mental health nurse with a wide range of clinical experience spanning more than 20 years. In addition to her university work she is a professional musician and does voluntary work for various mental health organisations including being the coordinator for the Hampshire Human Library – an international initiative aimed at reducing stigma through interaction and education of the public. She is the creative director of The Sanity Company which publishes books aimed at helping children and young people develop good mental health and problem-solving skills.

Janine Ward

Janine Ward is an accredited Psychological Wellbeing Practitioner (PWP) and Mental Health Practitioner by background and has worked within forensic mental health, learning difficulties, community mental health and substance abuse teams. Janine currently team leads the Southampton Improving Access to Psychological Therapies Low Intensity and Assessment Team and provides some clinical leadership across her employing Trust. She is seconded as a PWP educator at the University of Southampton and has worked within the Health Sciences Faculty for the last three years. Janine is currently studying for her PhD at Southampton.

Foreword

In mental healthcare there has been an explosion in psychosocial interventions over the last 15 years with a dizzying array of therapies and techniques being employed. Add this to the complexity of human beings, operating from a comprehensive array of cultural backgrounds and beliefs; various levels of knowledge and understanding; differing likes and dislikes, life experience and behaviours and you have a highly complex and often confusing mix. Considering this situation a guide to some of the techniques we can employ to help is called for.

If you were training to be a plumber you would expect to be introduced to the tools of the trade and given instruction in how to use them. This book is a toolkit of some of those interventions you may find useful in your practice designed with exercises and real life applications that will help equip you for your career in caring for others. There are frequent calls within the book for you to practice these skills yourself and employ the techniques within your own lives. Many of these interventions are also useful life skills and using them in your own life will not only help you to develop yourself, it will also put you in a position of deeper understanding with those you care for as you will understand some of the difficulties in changing behaviours first hand. A good axiom here is not to ask others to do things we would not be happy to do ourselves.

There are two additional issues that are of particular note in order to ensure you are practising safely and effectively. The first is, do not imagine that reading this book, or doing a short course in many of the techniques within, makes you an expert in that therapeutic approach. Most therapies take training, time and practice to become proficient in. Do be clear however, that there are many interventions inherent in those therapeutic approaches that can be usefully employed in collaboration with the service user to help them on their journey to recovery. The second point is to remember at all times to be guided by the people you care for as to the different priorities for intervention. All too often service users complain they are not listened to and that services have unrealistic expectations of them. If we want to help people to recover we must work with them in a collaborative way to ensure they are leading the changes, clear on the goals we are aiming for and help motivate them to succeed.

If you are a student nurse, a newly qualified nurse or even a nurse of some years standing looking for tips to update your portfolio of skills, this book will stand you in good stead for practice. It can be read as a whole but can also be dipped into section by section as you come across situations in practice, perhaps, that warrant further exploration of that particular subject. Engaging with this book will help you to become a more effective practitioner of the art of mental health nursing, enhancing your ability to facilitate recovery with people of diverse backgrounds and needs.

Sandra Walker

Acknowledgements

The publisher and authors wish to thank Chris Williams for permission to reproduce his 'Five Areas Model' from *Overcoming Depression and Low Mood*, 3rd edition, CRC Press 2009, which appears as 'A CBT model', Figures 2.1 and 2.2 in Chapter 2, and as Figures 5.1, 5.3, 5.4 and 5.6 in Chapter 5.

We also thank P.K. Gordon for permission to reproduce the Emotions Wheel (as Figure 5.5 in Chapter 5) available from www.getselfhelp.co.uk.

Introduction

Who is this book for?

This book is written primarily for student nurses currently undertaking their pre-qualification training. It will also be useful for junior nurses who are just beginning their careers and would be a useful refresher for anyone who regularly cares for people in mental distress.

Why *Psychosocial Interventions*?

Psychosocial interventions include a range of techniques that can help us care effectively for people without the risk of unwanted side-effects or negative consequences. In order to provide truly holistic healthcare we must know about the whole of a patient's life, not only the physical and psychological but also the social and spiritual aspects. In order to help someone recover it is important that we know how their lives are being impacted by their mental health and help them take action accordingly. In order to help us do this effectively we need a broad understanding of psychosocial interventions as well as drug treatments. While you would not expect to undertake any of the more formal therapies described here without training, there are aspects of them which can be applied in everyday mental healthcare. This book outlines some of the most commonly used interventions and provides ample information for you to explore further and practise some of these techniques.

Book structure

In Chapter 1, psychosocial interventions are defined and their role in effective, person-based and effective mental health care is discussed. The reader is given opportunities to consider mental health care within a psychosocial framework and clarify the theoretical underpinnings of psychosocial interventions. Additionally we consider the challenges of delivering psychosocial interventions in routine mental health care.

Chapter 2 considers cognitive behavioural therapy (CBT) more closely, seeking to understand the development of CBT as a therapeutic intervention, describe and explain the key components of using a CBT model for assessment of problems and critically consider the use of tools to aid in both assessment and treatment monitoring. The structure of a CBT session is considered, to ensure effective use of time and resources in a therapeutic context and there are important opportunities to reflect on your own experience of using some of the tools available in CBT.

In Chapter 3 we look at dialectical behavioural therapy (DBT), another form of therapy in order to help us to understand the components of a DBT programme and its aims. There are suggestions regarding the patient groups for whom DBT may prove an effective treatment, a description of the skills used in a DBT programme and how these may be used. Additionally you have the opportunity to practise DBT skills within you own daily life, reinforcing how important it is that you believe in the skills when supporting a patient to learn and practise them. The chapter ends with a discussion of how to support a patient undertaking a DBT programme.

Mindfulness, an ancient technique now regularly used in mental health practice is explained in Chapter 4, looking at the concept of mindfulness and the benefits that it may have for people practising the technique. There is some discussion regarding which patient groups it may be useful for, along with a more practical element whereby the author describes how to perform an activity or exercise mindfully. We then move on to evaluate a variety of different mindfulness exercises from experience and discuss some of the difficulties people may have when learning mindfulness and how these may be overcome. Finally, the role of the nurse in working alongside patients learning and practising mindfulness techniques is considered.

Chapter 5 considers low intensity interventions concentrating on low intensity CBT, behavioural activation, cognitive restructuring, exposure therapy and problem-solving therapy. Each intervention is considered mainly in the light of anxiety in order to create a useful framework of reference to bring the theory to life.

In Chapter 6 the importance of physical activity as a psychosocial intervention is considered. The reader is asked to critically evaluate the policy surrounding physical activity and demonstrate knowledge of the evidence base around the benefits of physical activity. The chapter will enable you to better understand the levels of activity that are necessary to benefit both mental and physical health and suggest strategies to help your patients become more active while also highlighting some of the cautions to physical activity.

Chapter 7, our final chapter here, considers the complex issues of dual diagnosis, mental health and the interplay with substance misuse. While the different expressions of dual diagnosis in all fields of nursing are described, the focus is to help the reader to understand common relationships between mental health and substance use. The perceptions of the dual diagnosis patient group are considered along with information regarding some of the treatments available.

Requirements for the NMC *Standards for Pre-registration Nursing Education* and the *Essential Skills Clusters*

The Nursing and Midwifery Council (NMC) has established standards of competence to be met by applicants to different parts of the register, and these are the standards it considers necessary for safe and effective practice. In addition to the competencies, the NMC has set out specific skills that nursing students must be able to perform at various points of an education programme. These are known as Essential Skills Clusters (ESCs). This book is structured so that it will help you to understand and meet the competencies and ESCs required for entry to the NMC register. The relevant competencies and ESCs are presented at the start of each chapter so that you can clearly see which ones the chapter addresses. There are *generic standards* that all nursing students irrespective of their field must achieve, and *field-specific standards* relating to each field of nursing, i.e. mental health, children's, learning disability and adult nursing. Most chapters have generic standards, and mental health field-specific standards are also listed.

This book includes the latest standards for 2010 onwards, taken from 'Standards for pre-registration nursing education' (NMC, September 2010).

Learning features

Throughout the book you will find activities in the text that will help you to make sense of, and learn about, the material being presented by the authors.

Some activities ask you to reflect on aspects of practice, or your experience of it, or the people or situations you encounter. *Reflection* is an essential skill in nursing, and it helps you to understand the world around you and often to identify how things might be improved. Other activities will help you develop key skills such as your ability to *think critically* about a topic in order to challenge received wisdom, or your ability to *research a topic and find appropriate information and evidence*, and to be able to make decisions using that evidence in situations that are often difficult and time-pressured. Finally, communication and working as part of a team are core to all nursing practice, and some activities will ask you to carry out *group activities* or think about your *communication skills* to help develop these.

All the activities require you to take a break from reading the text, think through the issues presented and carry out some independent study, possibly using the internet. Where appropriate, there are sample answers presented at the end of each chapter, and these will help you to understand more fully your own reflections and independent study. Remember, academic study will always require independent work; attending lectures will never be enough to be successful on your programme, and these activities will help to deepen your knowledge and understanding of the issues under scrutiny and give you practice at working on your own.

You might want to think about completing these activities as part of your personal development plan (PDP) or portfolio. After completing the activity write it up in your PDP or portfolio in a section devoted to that particular skill, then look back over time to see how far you are developing. You can also do more of the activities for a key skill that you have identified a weakness in, which will help build your skill and confidence in this area.

It is the aim of this book to have an interactive style using realistic scenarios, to be a book that explains how, as well as why, whilst taking account of the complexity of modern healthcare, thereby providing the reader with practical tools to add to their toolbox of skills to assist those we care for on their road to recovery.

Chapter 1
An introduction to psychosocial interventions

Wendy Turton

NMC Standards for Pre-registration Nursing Education

Domain 1: Professional values

4.1   Mental health nurses must work with people in a way that values, respects and explores the meaning of their individual lived experiences of mental health problems, to provide person-centred and recovery-focused practice.

5.   All nurses must fully understand the nurse's various roles, responsibilities and functions, and adapt their practice to meet the changing needs of people, groups, communities and populations.

Domain 2: Communication and interpersonal skills

Mental health nurses must practise in a way that focuses on the therapeutic use of self. They must draw on a range of methods of engaging with people of all ages experiencing mental health problems, and those important to them, to develop and maintain therapeutic relationships. They must work alongside people, using a range of interpersonal approaches and skills to help them explore and make sense of their experiences in a way that promotes recovery.

5.   All nurses must use therapeutic principles to engage, maintain and, where appropriate, disengage from professional caring relationships, and must always respect professional boundaries.

5.1   Mental health nurses must use their personal qualities, experiences and interpersonal skills to develop and maintain therapeutic, recovery-focused relationships with people and therapeutic groups. They must be aware of their own mental health, and know when to share aspects

NMC Essential Skills Clusters (ESCs)

Cluster: Care, compassion and communication

6.   People can trust the newly registered graduate nurse to engage therapeutically and actively listen to their needs and concerns, responding using skills that are helpful, providing information that is clear, accurate, meaningful and free from jargon.

By entry to the register:

7. Consistently shows ability to communicate safely and effectively with people providing guidance for others.
8. Communicates effectively and sensitively in different settings, using a range of methods and skills.

Chapter aims

After reading this chapter, you will be able to:

- define what psychosocial interventions (PSIs) are and their role in effective, person-based mental health care;
- provide opportunities to consider mental health care within a psychosocial framework;
- clarify the theoretical underpinnings of PSIs;
- consider the challenges of delivering PSIs in routine mental health care.

Introduction: psychosocial interventions

Case study

Marianne lives with recurrent depression and this time round has been off sick from her job for five months; this latest episode of low mood has caused her to become anxious about returning to work; she has lost confidence in herself and wonders how she will cope with the inevitable questions from her work colleagues. Marianne received a comprehensive psychosocial package of care from her mental health team. Working alongside Marianne, her care team identified that to promote and sustain recovery, she needed appropriate but minimal medication to support her mood. This was as an adjunct to a course of CBT for her depression, to enable Marianne to understand her vulnerability to depression and learn skills to prevent relapsing into a further episode. Marianne's husband received support from the carer's support worker so that he could understand more about depression and so be a pivotal support for Marianne's recovery. Vocational support was given to Marianne and her employer's HR department to support a staggered return to her workplace and Marianne received support with accessing the local leisure centre to begin increasing her level of exercise. Lastly, Marianne was also supported to access bibliotherapy to develop her confidence in managing her mood vulnerability and well-being. Marianne has been discharged for two years now and has not experienced a relapse into depression.

Psychosocial interventions are a group of non-pharmacological therapeutic interventions which address the psychological, social, personal, relational and vocational problems associated with mental health disorders. Psychosocial interventions address both the primary symptoms of the mental health problem and the secondary experiences which arise as a consequence of the mental health problem; as such PSIs are a person-based intervention rather than a solely symptom-based treatment. There are many different therapeutic models and techniques that fall under the umbrella of PSIs such as cognitive behavioural therapy (CBT), dialectical behavioural therapy (DBT), supported employment, and peer support, and we will return to these different techniques and models later in the chapter; some are termed psychological *therapies* but they do come under the PSI umbrella.

The PSIs offered to the person experiencing mental health difficulties will depend on the type of problem they are experiencing and their comprehensive needs, taking into account the impact that the mental health problem has had on their lives. Psychosocial interventions take an overview of the person's unique situation, which is why a comprehensive and collaborative assessment process is necessary. Interagency working is also necessary because the various forms of PSI offered to the individual may come from a number of different sources. For example, someone experiencing psychosis and living with their family may be offered cognitive behavioural family interventions work (CBFI), while someone living with emotionally unstable personality disorder may be offered DBT; both may be offered vocational or educational support and possibly peer support with a view to reducing isolation. The choice is supported through the evidence base for the various therapies and interventions and the findings which support efficacy of the interventions. Following systematic review of available evidence, the National Institute for Health and Care Excellence (NICE) Guidelines for various mental health disorders also recommend specific PSIs.

No matter what model or technique is utilised, the aim of PSIs is to promote, support and maintain recovery by providing:

- a framework for a comprehensive and meaningful assessment ensuring all elements of experience which are pertinent to promoting and maintaining recovery are covered;
- support which is meaningful and psychotherapeutic;
- a framework for developing a bio-psychosocial understanding of the person's experience, developed collaboratively with the person;
- psychological interventions which reduce distress;
- psychological therapy to explore personal psychological vulnerabilities which leave a person open to ongoing mental health problems;
- psychosocial interventions which reduce the interference the mental health difficulties have on the person's life;
- support to reconnect with the social world and so reduce the deleterious impact of social exclusion and isolation;
- support to consider educational and employment opportunities;
- support to regain or develop skills which assist in self-care and activities of daily life;
- cognitive remediation to enhance concentration and cognitive processes.

Case study

Chelsea is 29 years old. Chelsea dropped out of school when she was 15 and spent three years 'sofa surfing' with friends to avoid sleeping at home. Chelsea was sexually abused by two of her mum's short-term partners when she was 8 and 14, and emotionally abused and neglected by her mum over many years. Chelsea found employment in various cafés and takeaways and has thrown away her dream of going to university and making something of her life. Chelsea was finally re-housed by the council but ten years on, finds her life can still be chaotic. She has been self-harming by cutting since she was 9, and has had periods when she minimised this and times when she was self-harming frequently. She has moved the body area of cutting so that it is not visible to her customers and her employers. People at work view her as bubbly, if more than a little 'crazy'; she is very impulsive and can fly off the handle sometimes. They also note that Chelsea's mood is very changeable from extremes of happiness to morose-ness and anger, often triggered by the slightest of things. At home Chelsea often becomes distraught and uses alcohol to help her cope with her feelings. She does not cope well with endings or change, and is frequently lost in self-loathing and often feels alone and misunderstood. The friends she makes seem to drift away when they get to know her and Chelsea believes this is because they see her as damaged; the truth is more that they find her inconsistent mood and behaviour difficult to tolerate. Just recently her latest boyfriend has ended their relationship because of her 'moods'. Chelsea finally agrees that she needs some help to change the way she gets through her life and her GP refers her to the Mental Health Assessment Team who accept the referral.

Activity 1.1   *Critical thinking*

What would a comprehensive assessment with Chelsea reveal in terms of her needs and what areas might we need to consider addressing in order to promote sustainable change in Chelsea?

An outline answer to this activity is provided at the end of the chapter.

PSIs have gained momentum over the past two decades because of the growing recognition of psychological processes in the development and maintenance of common and more severe mental health problems. Equally more and more evidence informs us that social isolation, societal stigma and self-stigma are common experiences for people experiencing mental health problems and can impede recovery. We know the havoc mental health problems can wreak on all aspects of a person's life, and that merely reducing symptoms will not create a holistic recovery. The strengthening position of the recovery movement in mental health has also supported the fostering of treatment regimens based on PSI rather than a reliance on medication alone.

The psychosocial dimension

Sometimes in mental health we feel manoeuvred into taking a narrow perspective on people's recovery and find ourselves moving people on from mental health services when biological treatments appear to have stabilised the current health crisis; this situation means that the wider ramifications of a period of mental ill health are not addressed. The psychosocial dimension includes relapse prevention, our sense of ourselves, our aspirations, our relationships, employment, education, social inclusion, our ability to live independently and healthily, our sense of security in our world, our physical health and many more.

Activity 1.2   *Reflection*

Dimensions of our lives

Reflect on how many aspects of your life there are, what roles you take in your life, what responsibilities, pleasures, stresses and aspirations you have.

Imagine yourself experiencing high levels of anxiety; reflect on how living with this anxiety would impact and compromise your current life. What difficulties would it create? What might you not be able to continue doing? What might you lose because of the anxiety?

Every health problem has a psychosocial dimension so recovery must be supported within this dimension concurrently with any appropriate pharmacological and physiological treatments. Psychosocial interventions are not in essence anti-pharmacological, but are equally effective as pharmacological treatment in some disorders, e.g. depression (NICE, 2009) and are recommended as concurrent interventions with pharmacological treatments in other disorders, e.g. psychosis (NCCMH, 2014). The best treatment regimens use both in parallel, ensuring that the psychosocial intervention is delivered in a professional and ethical manner and the medication is prescribed at the minimum efficacious dose; such concurrent treatments can arguably increase self-agency in recovery.

Mental health nursing and psychosocial interventions

PSIs are a central element of a mental health nurse's role. Your key skills are comprehensive and collaborative assessment of a person's mental health needs, knowing the recommendations for efficacious intervention in mental health problems, gaining clinical skills in some of the psychosocial therapies used in treatment, and understanding the importance of the psychosocial domain in treatment and recovery. Care co-ordination itself supports a psychosocial approach to intervention because such a holistic approach needs a central person to co-ordinate the range of interventions that are appropriate and to signpost or refer to other agencies.

Case study

Derek is 46 years old. Derek has never married but had a steady long-term job with the local council and a healthy social network mostly with his friends from work. During his life Derek has had a number of short-lived episodes of low mood which he says went away with getting stuck into work, having a short holiday, supported by taking a short course of anti-depressants. He moved to Hampshire five years ago to be nearer to his elderly mother after the death of his father. Since moving

---

to Hampshire Derek has been the main carer for his mum, whilst struggling to hold down a job with the local council. Nine months ago Derek hurt his back whilst decorating and has been in constant pain since then. He is on long-term sick leave from work but is now on Statutory Sick Benefit and struggling financially. Derek reported to his GP that his mood has lowered again, but that there is nothing that can bring it back up. Derek feels as if his life is a failure, he cannot work, cannot look after his mum, and has no respite from his worries and racing thoughts. He feels despairing and pessimistic. He feels trapped, lonely and hopeless.

Activity 1.3 — *Team working*

As a care co-ordinator, identify the psychosocial needs that Derek has. What other agencies and professional disciplines might you need to involve in this care? How would you co-ordinate the range of PSIs indicated as appropriate in Derek's holistic recovery-led care?

An outline answer to this activity is provided at the end of the chapter.

Training and expert clinical supervision are a must to support PSI delivery. When we as nurses identify that a PSI is appropriate for someone's treatment we must ensure that it is delivered at an appropriately high standard and that the quality of the intervention is rigorously monitored. Some forms of PSI require more training than others; CBT and DBT (two of the psychological therapies under the PSI umbrella) for example require professionally led clinical training followed by structured clinical supervision, whereas PSIs that focus on employment or educational needs will have a different training and supervision structure, and some PSIs such as using a cognitive behavioural approach to intervention can be supported through less intense training and good supervision – but using this approach for example is not the same as delivering CBT, and it is important that we know what we are delivering and are aware of the limitations of our knowledge and skills. It is equally important that we do not undertake to deliver PSIs that we do not thoroughly understand or have not received appropriate training for, particularly so when we are considering the psychological therapies.

Theoretical underpinnings of psychosocial interventions: the stress-vulnerability model

Psychosocial interventions are underpinned by the stress-vulnerability model of health; it is important that we spend some time in this introductory chapter familiarising ourselves with this key concept.

Whilst there were earlier writers developing the stress-vulnerability model, Zubin and Spring offered a seminal paper on this model in 1977 focusing particularly on psychosis, and other writers have continued the development of the model since and considered it as a framework for wider psychopathology (e.g. Nuechterlein and Dawson, 1984; Ingram and Luxton, 2005). Within this model both the impact of stress on the individual and their predisposing vulnerabilities are recognised determinants of health. In mental health, this model supports the understanding that all of us have particular biological and psychological vulnerabilities to developing mental health problems or illnesses when combined with a 'critical' amount of stress in our lives. Indeed, the understanding of the interaction of stress and vulnerability is arguably essential for understanding the development of mental health problems (Ingram and Luxton, 2005).

Nuechterlein and Dawson (1984) proposed that enduring vulnerability plus stress leads to a transient intermediate state of a cognitive, interpersonal and intrapersonal processing overload which leads to 'outcome behaviour'. They specifically looked at psychosis and so deemed the outcome behaviour to be the symptoms of psychosis, but we can extrapolate from their modelling to other mental health disorders, whereby personal vulnerability plus stress lead to a similar overload which results in anxiety disorders or depression, self-harming behaviour, 'behaviour that challenges', or another expression of mental distress. 'Behaviours that challenge' is a term in the mental health field which describes 'actions and incidents that may, or have potential to, physically or psychologically harm another person or self, or property' (SA Health, 2012)

How do we define stress?

Stress is an accessible lay concept; we can each quite readily recognise stress by reflecting on our own lives. Stressors, those elements of our life which cause us to experience stress, can be significant life events; for example one highly significant event, a traumatic experience, a major life change, a personal loss. But stress can also be a culmination of minor life stressors which add up to a major stressful impact on our life and so on our health, both mental and physical.

It is important to note that stressors can be external or internal. External stressors are, as noted, easily identified. But how do we account for individual differences in response to common stressors? The answer is that the very manner in which we perceive and then appraise the stressor is dependent on our own cognitive and psychological make-up. Some of us may find particular life events easier to cope with because we do not view them as a significant threat to our psychological or physiological integrity; we do not see them as insurmountable, life changing, challenging, or bringing with them serious personal consequences. We have a sense that we are capable of managing the particular stressors; we either are confident in our personal resources or have a supportive network to help us cope. But others of us will see the same stressor as being more threatening or consequential, and more perhaps we do not have the same 'coping' styles, so that we make a different appraisal of the stressor and that determines our response to it.

Experiencing stress impacts on our wellbeing because it disrupts our usual ways of coping with our lives. Stress upsets both our physiological and psychological processes, changing our thought processes, our emotions, and the way our body responds. Our immune system can become compromised because of this impact causing us to be more physically vulnerable to ill health, and stress hormones such as adrenaline and cortisol can impact on other physiological systems such as our blood pressure and our digestive system, causing further problems.

Ways that we would normally manage our lives become compromised, and those strategies familiar to us for coping become inaccessible or useless. We probably find ourselves not coping as well as we usually would, behaving in unfamiliar ways, and instead of managing the difficulties that have arisen we find that we are overwhelmed and disabled by the stress, often stuck in attempts to manage the stress which inadvertently maintain our stressful experience rather than alleviate it. Over time stress becomes distress, and our lives and our mental health become more seriously impacted.

How do we define vulnerability?

Vulnerability is defined as a predispositional factor that makes us more likely to respond to stress in particular ways and so more likely to develop problematic mental health states. Vulnerabilities are biological, genetic and psychological. Biological and genetic factors are stable and usually latent factors within a person's make-up, which become known when a critical mass of stress is experienced. Vulnerability to psychosis is often the case that is given as an example. Whilst the aetiology (cause) of psychosis is not certain, there is evidence that suggests a biological or genetic vulnerability for the development of this disorder, which is latently but enduringly present within the individual, only developing as a mental health illness following the experience of personally significant levels of stress (Zubin and Spring, 1977; Nuechterlein and Dawson, 1984). Psychological vulnerabilities can stem from faulty learning (Ingram and Luxton, 2005) or exposure to traumatic or abusive events during earlier years (Lanktree and Briere, 2008), including from dysfunctional attachment to primary care givers (Gumley et al., 2014). Vulnerabilities are now robustly argued to include reduced cognitive processing capacity, autonomic hypersensitivity, and interpersonal and personal skill deficits including poor emotional literacy, and equally robustly shown to be linked to mental health problems (Ingram and Price, 2010).

The important factor about biological and psychological vulnerability factors is that they are accessible to treatment and so to change. For example, autonomic hypersensitivity, a biological vulnerability which is linked to anxiety disorders, is responsive to medication and to psychological interventions (Anxiety Care UK, 2014). Psychological vulnerabilities are highly responsive to PSIs.

Vulnerabilities can be defined as proximal or distal factors. Distal vulnerability factors, meaning further away from the onset of the mental health problem, might include developmental experiences which were aversive to normal development, and perhaps developed in us low self-esteem, or a view of the world of being threatening and untrustworthy. Proximal vulnerability factors, meaning closer to the development of the mental health problem, might be the thinking styles or coping strategies which we have developed for managing stress, but which are influenced by our distal vulnerabilities and so not necessarily helpful strategies for resilience and stable mental health. Both types of vulnerability play a role in the development and maintenance of mental health disorders and both are amenable to change through PSIs (Ingram et al., 2011; Beck, 1976; Beck et al., 1979).

The convergence of stress and vulnerability

The stress-vulnerability model perceives mental health problems emerging as vulnerabilities and stresses converge and become too great a task for the individual to manage.

We all have a particular vulnerability to developing some form of mental distress given our 'critical' amount of stress. We probably do not know in advance what form that distress might take, nor will we be aware what our maximum capacity for stress will be. However, we will all be somewhere on the vulnerability axis depending on our early experiences and our biological and psychological make-up. Then, as our lives go along we will inevitably experience stress; the more stress, the higher up the stress axis we move. At a critical convergence of stress levels and vulnerability we will reach and go beyond the 'distress' line. Beyond this line, our vulnerabilities cause us to not have sufficient capacity to cope with the stresses, and our strengths and natural coping mechanisms are insufficient to manage the distress caused by our life stressors. It is at this point we begin to experience disordered emotional states which drive responsive behaviours; for some this will be an anxiety disorder, for others psychosis, for others depression. For some it will be expressed as self-harming behaviour or 'behaviours that challenge'. Figure 1.1 is a common and simplified depiction of this model.

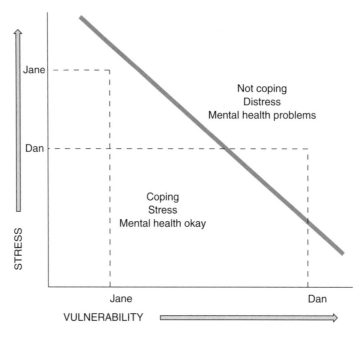

Figure 1.1: The stress-vulnerability model

We can see from Figure 1.1 above that when we use this model to understand the development of mental health distress we can visualise the convergence of stress and vulnerability and the development of psychological and emotional states which are beyond our capacity to manage.

We all have a level of vulnerability to developing mental health difficulties, we all have a limit to the amount of stress we can manage, we all have a 'critical point' when stress and vulnerability meet, and we can all cross the line into not coping, distress and mental health difficulties. None of us is absolutely aware of our vulnerabilities, and neither our ability to cope with life stresses. We do not know where our 'critical point' is, where we will cross the line in non-coping and distress (see Figure 1.1), nor do we know how our distress will be expressed; it may be anxiety, depression, psychosis or behaviours driven by an underlying personality disorder.

If we consider Jane from Figure 1.1, we can see that she has a fairly low vulnerability to developing mental health problems and so can manage a high amount of stress with lower consequences on her mental health. Dan, however, has a higher vulnerability to developing mental health problems and so it takes less life stress to move him across the line to distress and mental health difficulties.

Take some time to practise explaining this model of understanding mental health. The more familiar you are with this model the more confident you will feel when explaining it to service users.

Using psychosocial interventions informed by the stress-vulnerability model

We develop an understanding of a person's episode of mental health difficulties by assessing for present stressors, vulnerability factors and psychological make-up. We need to know what problems they are experiencing in their lives at this time (stressors), how they are appraising these difficulties (psychological make-up) and whether there are significant past events which have contributed to their current appraisal (vulnerabilities). That is, are there significant past events which influence the way they are reacting to their current stresses? We also need to know about strengths, both internal, e.g. cognitive styles, and external, e.g. social support. Psychosocial interventions aim to address the distress experienced by the person and the consequent disruption to life, so it is important that we gather information both about the level of subjective distress and about how people's lives have changed since the onset of their mental distress. This gives us a baseline for recovery and identifies therapeutic goals. When we have this information we are in a position to decide which PSIs will be most appropriate to promote and support recovery in that person.

Case study

Nicki is just 17 years old; her early life was troubled due to the tempestuous relationship between her parents. The father was gaoled for serious domestic violence when Nicki was 7 and she has not had any contact with him since. She has few friends at college as her experience of school has not been a happy one and she finds it difficult to trust her peers. Nicki has experienced ongoing bullying from a group of girls at her secondary school, including two incidents of physical harm from the group, one of which was filmed and posted online which caused Nicki to feel publicly humiliated. For a long time Nicki felt low and scared but recently has found a group of friends outside of the college who appear to accept her for who she is. Nicki has begun to spend most evenings and weekends with her new friends. They mostly hang around in the park, not causing trouble, but do smoke a lot of cannabis and dabble in other drugs. Nicki was beginning to feel happier, but suddenly finds herself feeling anxious again

(continued)

continued ... •

> *and a little paranoid, and now is aware that she is hearing a voice that no one else can hear. Nicki is worried because her Uncle David has had quite severe mental health problems all his life, so finally she confides in her mum. Nicki reluctantly attends a GP appointment with her mum and is referred to the Adult Mental Health Services.*

Activity 1.4	*Critical thinking*

If Nicki was offered only anti-psychotic medication, what would be missed in promoting a holistic and sustainable recovery?

An outline answer to this activity is provided at the end of the chapter.

The importance of a stress-vulnerability approach to mental health

This understanding of psychopathology affords us as nurses a valuable opportunity to intervene therapeutically and meaningfully. It defines mental health disorders as consisting of domains (stress and vulnerability) which are understandable and accessible to biological, psychological and social interventions. Let us consider depression: we know that certain early events and life experiences make us more vulnerable to developing depression given our critical stress capacity, and we have evidence that biological (medication and exercise), psychological and social interventions are effective in promoting and maintaining recovery (NCCMH, 2010). Our practice is therefore guided by using this stress vulnerability framework to help develop a collaborative understanding of the development and maintenance of the depression, the identification of strengths and of underdeveloped skills, and the use of PSIs to address recovery through addressing psychological vulnerabilities and both internal and external stressors.

Case study

If we think back to Derek, we are not sure from the information we begin with about what has caused Derek to be vulnerable to developing depression when life stresses become unmanageable, so our journey would begin with exploring his life experiences and his psychological make-up to better determine what his vulnerabilities are. We also need to know what stresses he is able to cope with without experiencing low mood, and those which trigger low mood. We are aware that he has had a previous strategy for coping with his mood change, which seemed to work for him. We need to assess what is different for him now that is causing his previous coping strategies to be less effective. For Derek, triggers for this episode of low mood are likely to be internal as well as external. We know that he is managing a great deal of stress from his current life circumstances and that there are many depressogenic factors around for Derek such as many losses in recent times (father, old work mates, old role in life, physical ability, financial security). We also know that people with recurrent depression can experience relapse because there is an overreaction to negative thoughts and short-term low mood, fuelling a relapse into depression. Thus, we need to engage Derek in an exploration of vulnerabilities, current stresses, previous strengths and what is causing these previous strategies not to work now. We can develop an understanding of those strategies and explanations we need to develop in Derek to help promote and sustain his recovery this time.

We might for example offer CBT to address the psychological depressogenic vulnerabilities and the internal stressors of negative thinking and we might offer psychosocial support through behavioural activation and increasing social contacts to address isolation and the withdrawal from opportunities offering positive feedback. There may too be issues of employment support and support increase in physical exercise, as well as monitoring medication regimens.

What kinds of psychosocial interventions are there?

Many PSIs exist and their point of focus varies. Difficulties in life are never isolated to one issue, or exist only in one area; difficulties in one area impact on other areas of life. Being anxious will influence your relationships, how you are able to be with your friends, how you are able to remain in employment or not. A useful element of PSIs is that when we choose a target for treatment, benefits from that specific focus will ripple out into other areas of our lives that had become problematic. So we might focus on anxiety management, but through that focus you may be able to sustain a return to work or develop confidence in friendships again. Indeed the most effective PSIs encourage the recipient to extrapolate the learning from a specific focus of therapy to other areas of their life, thus allowing for the generalising of successful experiences, new learning and change. Psychosocial interventions are collaborative in nature and as such do require the use of good engagement skills to develop and support a commitment by the person to engaging with the intervention. The recipient is an active participant in any PSI, ultimately being left at the end of the PSI input with the skills to maintain and further promote their own recovery thereby increasing well-being and reducing the likelihood of relapse.

Table 1.1 indicates the types of interventions that can fall under the umbrella of PSI. Their range is wide because the psychosocial domain of our lives is diverse. Psychosocial life elements are also inter-related so that addressing one area will influence another. This can be illustrated for example when focusing on increasing social contacts for people living with psychosis in that this enhanced relational aspect of their lives can impact positively on self-esteem and improved mood.

Cognitive behaviour therapy	Group interventions	Physical health monitoring
Mindfulness-based cognitive therapy	Independent living skills	
	Coping strategy enhancement	Lifestyle education
Dialectical behavioural therapy		Vocational support
Acceptance and commitment therapy	Health education	Peer support
	Cognitive remediation	Spiritual support
Compassion-focused therapy	Computer-assisted therapy	Social support
Schema-focused therapy	Self-help	Social skills training
Psychodynamic counselling	Bibliotherapy	Social inclusion
Family interventions		

Table 1.1: Interventions under the PSI umbrella

Descriptions of some psychosocial interventions

Here are some brief explanations of a few PSIs to begin to develop your understanding and knowledge; the book will of course cover some in depth.

Cognitive behavioural therapy

Cognitive behavioural therapy is a psychological therapy developed by Aaron Beck in the 1960s. This model explores the sense we make of events (our thoughts), how unhelpful thoughts and thinking styles are associated with troublesome emotional and physiological states, and drive behaviours which maintain our problems rather than resolve them. CBT has a robust evidence base across many mental health disorders. To deliver the therapy, specialist training is required. Traditional CBT is termed 'second wave' CBT.

Third wave cognitive therapies are those CBT-based therapies which do not work to challenge thoughts but focus on acceptance of the troublesome or distressing thought and a non-reactive acknowledgement of them.

Cognitive behavioural family interventions

Cognitive behavioural family interventions are supported in the NICE Guideline for the treatment of psychosis (NCCMH, 2014) for all individuals experiencing psychosis who remain in contact with their families. This therapy works with the whole family unit to explore the problems associated with the presence of psychosis within the family unit. It uses collaborative approaches to distress and problem minimisation through enhancing understanding and communication within the family.

Mindfulness-based cognitive therapy

A third wave cognitive therapy using mindfulness-based cognitive therapy (MBCT) as a therapeutic technique (Segal et al., 2002). Mindfulness is a form of meditation which allows for an awareness of distressing emotional arousal or problematic cognitive processes to be gained by the person and then to apply a meditative approach to managing and changing that response or process. This therapy is developing an evidence base of effectiveness for both depression and psychosis.

Acceptance and commitment therapy

Acceptance and commitment therapy (ACT) is a 'third wave' cognitive therapy (Hayes and Strosahl, 2004) which focuses more on the behavioural component of a person's problematic experience, exploring the function of the behaviour rather than the content. ACT can be used transdiagnostically – that is that this is a PSI which is not linked specifically to the treatment of a particular diagnosable mental health condition but can be used for a variety of psychologically distressing experiences whatever the underlying cause.

Person-based cognitive therapy

Person-based cognitive therapy (PBCT; Chadwick, 2006) is another third wave cognitive therapy, used specifically for people who hear distressing voices.

Dialectical behaviour therapy

Dialectical behaviour therapy (Linehan, 1993a) is a further third wave therapy which is designed for working with people who have specific personality disorders.

Psychodynamic counselling

Psychodynamic counselling works through the present to access the past which is believed to influence us in the present but perhaps outside our consciousness. This allows for exploration of subconscious conflicts within ourselves that are keeping us stuck in our present problematic and distressing circumstances. Psychodynamic counselling can be used for a broad range of issues including relationships, anxiety, depression, trauma and abuse.

Bibliotherapy

Bibliotherapy uses books to treat mild mental health problems. People can be helped by reading appropriate 'self-help' material. Books are now available covering a wide range of subjects including anxiety, bereavement, depression, self-esteem and stress. Such books are usually written by field experts and offer explanations, first person accounts and practical tips. Bibliotherapy can be either supported or unsupported by a nurse or clinician. This style of intervention can be offered at any step in the care pathway from pre-primary care to secondary care.

Support groups

Support groups are therapeutic forums in which people who share similar experiences, problems or aims meet together to support each other in staying well. They can be facilitated by nurses and other professionals, or can be self-facilitated. Support groups can be created to support many problematic experiences and have an additional social context compared to individual support or therapy.

Computer-assisted therapy

Computer-assisted therapies have grown in number over the last few years due to the accessibility and increasing reliance on computer technology. They are special online learning packages similar but going beyond bibliotherapy. Like bibliotherapy, computer-assisted therapies can be facilitated by professionals or done alone. This type of therapy most often addresses depression but its range is widening particularly due to the increase in therapy 'apps' for smart phones.

Vocational support

Vocational services provide support and practical help for people with mental health problems who want to return to work. Support can be through individual support outside of the workplace or can be supporting someone during their return to work within the workplace and through negotiating with employers.

Creating an environment for psychosocial interventions in mental health care

Mental health service provision has been through radical changes over the past 40 years in the UK since the movement to close off large asylum-oriented care and embrace community-based care. There have been several reorganisations of NHS and social care services over these years, and variations in funding, but provision of mental health treatment continues to be under-resourced (LSE, 2012).

Back in 2007 there was an increased sense of optimism about NHS mental health service provision. The 2007 Appleby Report *Mental Health Ten Years On: Progress on Mental Health Care Reform* on the then Labour Government's ten year plan of mental health reform launched in 1999 noted an increase in mental health funding, major developments in community mental health teams with 100,000 people being treated at home rather than admitted to hospital and large increases in all the main staff groups, including a rise of 1300 consultant psychiatrists, 2700 clinical psychologists and almost 10,000 mental health nurses. The national patient survey at that time showed that 77 per cent of community patients rated their care as good, very good or excellent. The suicide rate had fallen to the lowest figure on record – and records began in 1861 – and the WHO said that England has the best mental health services in Europe.

This ten-year programme included the establishment of NICE to provide national guidance and advice to improve health and social care. These NICE Guidelines for best clinical practice provided recommendations for treatments based on a systematic review of research evidence, and such recommendations support the use of PSIs in mental health care.

The development of IAPT and the Stepped Model of Care

In 2008 the National IAPT (Increasing Access to Psychological Therapies) services were developed, providing evidence-based psychological and psychosocial treatments for people experiencing depression or anxiety disorders in primary care. IAPT services were developed around the Stepped

Model of Care (NICE, 2011) whereby care provided is initially the least intensive intervention that is appropriate for that person, and people can step up or down the care pathway as according to changed needs and in response to treatment. At present, Steps 1 to 3 are primary care and IAPT, Step 4 is community mental health care, and Step 5 is inpatient or equivalent intensive home treatment and specialist mental health services. What this does mean is that there is a provision of different PSIs depending in which Step people are accessing their mental health care.

IAPT is in an initial six-year expansion programme, fully-funded in the Governmental Spending Reviews and designed by 2014 to provide NICE-recommended psychosocial and psychological therapy in Steps 2 and 3 care services each year to 15 per cent of those in the general population suffering from depression or anxiety disorders with a target recovery rate of 50 per cent. IAPT services are developing further, 2013 onwards, to consider how to increase access to psychosocial and psychological therapy for people experiencing severe mental health problems such as psychosis, bipolar disorder and personality disorder. These are likely to include workforce development in Steps 4 and 5 so that this provision can be provided by mental health practitioners, including mental health nurses, in these services.

A continuing struggle

A change of UK Government in 2010 brought in superseding mental health policy documents beginning with the 2010 *Equity and Excellence: Liberating the NHS*, developing the role of NICE through their provision of quality standards for care. This was followed in 2011 by the *No Health without Mental Health* strategy with six shared objectives:

1. more people will have good mental health;
2. more people with mental health problems will recover;
3. more people with mental health problems will have good physical health;
4. more people will have a positive experience of care and support;
5. fewer people will suffer avoidable harm;
6. fewer people will experience stigma and discrimination.

However, in 2012 a report by the Mental Health Policy Group at the London School of Economics (LSE) *How Mental Illness Loses Out in the NHS* (LSE, 2012) noted that among people under 65, nearly half of all ill health is mental health illness, yet only a quarter of those are in treatment. They state:

> The under-treatment of people with crippling mental illnesses is the most glaring case of health inequality in our country.
> (p2)

In 2013 the UK Government published *Making Mental Health Services More Effective and Accessible* applicable to England NHS and social care services. The policy notes that the largest cause of disability in the UK remains poor mental health, and notes the link between poor mental health and a range of psychosocial problems such as employment, parenting, relationships, poor physical health and educational prospects. The aim of this latest policy is to force equality between mental and physical health services, make reducing mental health problems a priority for Public Health England, and include in these changes a further increase in the provision of psychological therapies.

Embracing an evidence-based treatment approach within mental health services should be the role of all mental health nurses, independently of the vagaries of Government. The potential annual savings to the NHS from the provision of interventions to treat depression for those currently untreated could be as high as £16 million by 2026 (King's Fund, 2008).

Psychosocial treatments are shown to be effective in promoting and maintaining recovery, and the ethos of mental health nurses is to promote and support recovery. More, there is a professional empowerment in being directly involved in the recovery process of service users and delivering PSIs as an adjunct to medication, and providing a comprehensive treatment package offering a different quality of recovery than a medication-only approach. Indeed the 2006 *From Values to Action: The Chief Nursing Officer's Review of Mental Health Nursing* made a series of recommendations as to how mental health nurses could best improve the care provided to people with mental health problems. It noted that mental health nurses should incorporate the broad principles of the Recovery Approach into every aspect of their practice, being positive about change and promoting social inclusion for mental health users and carers. There was also a focus on improving outcomes for service users underpinned by the principles of PSIs: positive therapeutic relationships, taking a holistic approach and providing more evidence-based psychological therapies. Embracing a psychosocial approach to mental health nursing care and availing ourselves of the range of PSIs is a good step forward for all, our service users and our profession.

Chapter summary

- Psychosocial interventions should be used in mental health care to support a comprehensive and person-based effective approach that promotes and sustains recovery.
- Psychosocial interventions are underpinned by a parsimonious theoretical understanding of the development and maintenance of mental health problems – that is, a theory which is able to be simple and accessible and acceptably or robustly explanatory.
- There are many interventions which fall under the psychosocial umbrella; comprehensive and collaborative assessment guides the choice.
- It is an intrinsic part of every mental health nurse's role to incorporate a psychosocial approach within their mental health nurse practice.

Activities: brief outline answers

Activity 1.1 Critical thinking

A comprehensive assessment might reveal the need for emotional coping skills or DBT.

Other areas to address might include: independent living skills, a return to education, psychological therapy to resolve trauma and vulnerability from her experience of recurrent abuse, relationship skill development, substance misuse education, assertive engagement to support Chelsea in committing to her care package.

Activity 1.3 Team working

Your answer might include: noting the major life change that Derek undertook five years ago, the reduction and loss of his social network, the increased burden of looking after his ailing mother, the loss of his father, his previous vulnerability to depression, current loneliness, financial pressures, employment insecurity, insecurity and possible pessimism about his future, ongoing physical ill-health, constant pain, depression. Agencies which could be part of a comprehensive psychosocial care package would include the mental health team, carer's support services, Derek's GP, physical health community teams, pain-management teams, physiotherapy, befriending services, peer support, social services to support the care for his mum. Co-ordination of such a complex inter-agency care package could be undertaken by the mental health care co-ordinator whilst Derek is under their care. This role would require good communication with Derek and all the agencies with an agreed format for sharing appropriate information. Aims and goals for this package of care, with agreed time scales for interventions, and agreed relationships with other agencies once Derek is discharged from mental health care are vital to prevent relapse and to support his sustained recovery from depression.

Activity 1.4 Critical thinking

Your answer might have included: psychological therapy to resolve the life traumas she has experienced which will act as a vulnerability to her future mental health, PSI to understand her potential increased vulnerability to developing psychosis and to strengthen her skills to minimise this potential outcome, relational and social literacy, substance misuse and its links to mental health problems and personal vulnerability to harm or exploitation from others, even for example the need for assertiveness training.

Further reading

Schizophrenia: Core Interventions in the Treatment and Management of Schizophrenia in Primary and Secondary Care (Update) [Internet]. Chapter 8. NICE Clinical Guidelines, No. 82. National Collaborating Centre for Mental Health (NCCMH), UK.

This chapter looks at psychological therapy and PSIs in the treatment and management of schizophrenia. It is available as an electronic book.

Mullen, A (2009) Mental health nurses establishing psychosocial interventions within acute inpatient settings. *International Journal of Mental Health Nursing*, 18(2): 83–9.

This article looks at the problems with mental health nursing practice in acute inpatient units, putting forward an argument for routine use of PSIs as a way of addressing some of these issues.

Smith, G (2012) *Psychological Interventions in Mental Health Nursing*. Berkshire: Open University Press.

This book provides further foundations in common psychological interventions used in mental health nursing.

Useful websites

www.bps.org.uk

The website of the British Psychological Society provides information and links to information about the use of psychology for the public good.

www.mind.org.uk/information-support/drugs-and-treatments/?gclid=COaq8cj7kb8CFUTItAoda WYAjA

MIND have a wealth of resources for mental health including information on PSIs which is written in clear language and especially useful for sharing with service users.

www.nice.org.uk/CG51

The National Institute for Health and Care Excellence website hosts a whole array of guidance designed to help us provide high quality care. This Clinical Guideline (51) outlines PSIs recommended for drug misuse.

Chapter 2
Cognitive behavioural therapy

Simon Grist

NMC Standards for Pre-registration Nursing Education

This chapter will address the following competencies:

Domain 3: Nursing practice and decision-making

4. All nurses must ascertain and respond to the physical, social and psychological needs of people, groups and communities. They must then plan, deliver and evaluate safe, competent, person-centred care in partnership with them, paying special attention to changing health needs during different life stages, including progressive illness and death, loss and bereavement.

4.1 Mental health nurses must be able to apply their knowledge and skills in a range of evidence-based psychological and psychosocial individual and group interventions to develop and implement care plans and evaluate outcomes, in partnership with service users and others.

8. All nurses must provide educational support, facilitation skills and therapeutic nursing interventions to optimise health and wellbeing. They must promote self-care and management whenever possible, helping people to make choices about their healthcare needs, involving families and carers where appropriate, to maximise their ability to care for themselves.

8.1 Mental health nurses must practise in a way that promotes the self-determination and expertise of people with mental health problems, using a range of approaches and tools that aid wellness and recovery and enable self-care and self-management.

Domain 4: Leadership, management and team working

4. All nurses must be self-aware and recognise how their own values, principles and assumptions may affect their practice. They must maintain their own personal and professional development, learning from experience, through supervision, feedback, reflection and evaluation.

4.1 Mental health nurses must actively promote and participate in clinical supervision and reflection, within a values-based mental health framework, to explore how their values, beliefs and emotions affect their leadership, management and practice.

Chapter aims

After reading this chapter you will be able to:

- understand the development of cognitive behavioural therapy (CBT) as a therapeutic intervention;
- describe and explain the key components of using a CBT model for assessment of problems;
- critically consider the use of tools to aid in both assessment and treatment monitoring that are both reliable and validated;
- consider the structure of a CBT session to ensure effective use of time and resources in a therapeutic context;
- reflect on your own experience of using some of the tools available in CBT.

What is CBT and how did it evolve?

Modern CBT, as we understand it, came predominantly from the work of Aaron Beck and Albert Ellis. The basic premise which underlies CBT can however be traced back to the Greek philosopher Epictetus (AD 55–135): *Men are disturbed not by things, but by the view that they take of them.*

This demonstrates one of the cornerstones of CBT: that the event itself, such as bereavement, job loss or marriage breakdown, is not key to how we react, but the belief behind the event is.

Activity 2.1   *Evidence-based practice and research*

Understanding the significance of the belief

Ask four or five of your friends to stand with their eyes closed. When they have closed their eyes tell them you are going to randomly pop a balloon in the room.

This will cause, hopefully, a range of reactions. Ask your friends what their thoughts were and why.

What you will see is that the situation was the same for everyone, however the reactions are likely to be different and the reason they are different is that the belief, or experience behind it, is the one that drives the reaction.

Modern CBT evolved from early work by psychologists such as Adler (1870–1937) whose ground-breaking work also reiterated the understanding that it is the meaning that we attach to events which is important. It was however the work of Bandura and Lazarus on thought processes that really began to form the basis of CBT that was picked up by Ellis and Beck in linking thought processes to outcomes, be they behavioural or cognitive.

CBT is the interaction of thoughts (cognitions), emotions, autonomic (physical) sensations and behaviour, which link and interact with each other (Padesky and Greenberger, 1995). By identification of these interacting systems CBT helps patients to make sense of how they process the world, and whether some of their behaviours and thought processes are maladaptive.

The role of the mental health nurse in CBT

CBT is increasingly being taken up by mental health nurses, and what used to be the domain of the psychologist is now increasingly becoming an additional role for nurses.

CBT is an evidence-based psychological intervention that ultimately allows patients to become better at understanding their responses to situations, when they are not helpful. It is focused on those who experience problems and offers a practical and easy to understand approach, allowing patients to make changes to their lives, and then to continue using these techniques to carry on improving the quality of their lives. It is therefore an intervention that sits well with mental health nurses and professionals; however, as a specific therapy it requires training. There are CBT courses available through most trusts and universities, as well as numerous private organisations. There is one governing body for those who wish to practise using CBT: the British Association of Behavioural and Cognitive Psychotherapists (BABCP) and it provides lists of accredited practitioners and training providers. This however does not stop a mental health nurse from using some of the principles to aid their understanding of a patient's problem and help in thinking about the right approach to take to help with this problem. However if you are using CBT techniques you should be supervised by a suitably qualified CBT practitioner.

The strongest evidence base for CBT is with patients suffering from anxiety and depression (National Institute for Health and Care Excellence (NICE), 2009, 2011). However CBT has been used to help patients suffering with substance use problems, chronic pain, schizophrenia and personality disorders to name a few. Since the establishment of the Improving Access to Psychological Therapies (IAPT) drive and recent Governmental White Papers (Talking Therapies, Department of Health (DH), 2011a), CBT has been growing in terms of its evidence base and application. Currently within mental health it is used across all settings; however this does not mean that all areas will have access to a CBT practitioner.

So, how does CBT work? It uses two psychological techniques to both help understand the problem and then to develop strategies to overcome the problem, or make it less acute.

Cognitive principles

The aim of cognitive processing is to examine clients' thoughts and help them learn the skill of recognising negative thoughts, often referred to as negative automatic thoughts (NATs). They will then be able re-evaluate these thoughts in an objective framework. This can involve using techniques to gather evidence for the validity of the thoughts, such as evidence for and against, surveys, or asking a trusted other person. Having done this, a client is then in a better position to evaluate the thought objectively and either create a more helpful thought, or be able to recognise the thought as unhelpful.

Activity 2.2   *Reflection*

Examining our own thoughts

Using a diary or a notebook keep a record of your negative thoughts for a couple of days. You do not need to show this to anyone, however make sure that you record all of your negative thoughts, no matter whether they caused you concern or not. Doing this allows you to have some understanding of the amount of negative thoughts that we all have daily. Why do you think we only record negative thoughts and not positive ones as well?

An outline answer to this activity is provided at the end of the chapter.

Behavioural principles

When patients feel anxious or depressed they often avoid doing activities, or they may exhibit behaviours that do not help them, although the patient will believe that the behaviour, or lack of, in some way protects them.

Case study

Richard had suffered with depression once before, but seemed to have naturally recovered from it. This episode, however, felt worse. He felt tired all of the time and had little motivation to go to work and see friends and felt hopeless about the future. He had been ringing into work to say that he was off sick and spending the day in bed. He did not feel hungry so was only eating a bit of toast in the evening. He felt that nobody could want to spend time with him as he was so useless and not much fun to be around. When his friends phoned him on the Friday evening to try and persuade him to go to the cinema he ignored the call. This made him feel better as he did not feel under pressure to go out and he knew that his friends would have a good time without him.

We will return to Richard later in the chapter.

Activity 2.3	*Critical thinking*

Identifying thoughts and behaviours

Write down all of the thoughts that Richard is having that could be considered negative. Then write down all of the behaviours that Richard is doing that he feels are helpful but we may feel are not.

An outline answer to this activity is provided at the end of the chapter.

Assessment and formulation using CBT

The process of using a CBT model involves collecting information from the patient across a number of areas. As we discussed earlier, CBT is the interaction of thoughts, emotions, physical sensations and behaviours. If we were to gather these generally across someone's life then the assessment would take a very long time! CBT is problem focused so we need to be specific and focus in on a particular problem, which then allows us to have a good depth of understanding around this problem.

Asking a patient to describe a recent episode when this problem was most prevalent allows us to be specific and allows the patient to give the detail required to help us to understand the problem. Using phrases such as 'can you tell me about the last time you felt like this?' or 'can you tell me what you were thinking and feeling when it happened' can be useful in allowing this detail to be gathered. We also want to ensure that we collect information around the four key areas of CBT (thoughts, emotions, physical sensations and behaviours) so we may have to ask specific questions to elicit responses from these domains. This is not a skill that can be taught after reading a chapter of a book; it takes practice and refinement. However, phrases such as 'what thoughts were going through your mind when it happened' or 'how did that make you feel?' allow us to guide the direction of the information to allow us to have a better understanding of the patient's experience.

| Activity 2.4 | *Evidence-based practice and research* |

Practising gathering information

With one of your peers have a go at collecting the information using a CBT model. Your peer needs to think of a recent situation where they have felt anxious or low (remembering to keep yourselves safe). Ask specific questions around the thoughts, emotions, physical sensations and behaviours to understand the nature of the problem.

How was that? Was any aspect of it easier than another? What made it easier to gather the information and how did your peer feel with your asking?

Using a 'hot cross bun model' such as Figure 2.1 may help you both gather the information and explain your perspective on this to the patient.

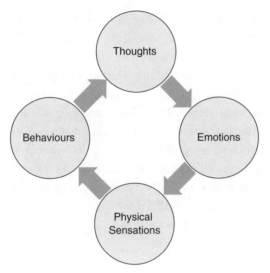

Figure 2.1: A CBT model

In CBT a collaborative stance is taken between practitioner and patient. This allows for a better working environment as the patient is the expert on their experience and you are the expert in the intervention (CBT) that is going to be used to help the patient to improve the quality of their life. It is therefore essential that you understand their problem in a way that makes sense for them, and aids with engagement as the patient feels 'understood'. Using the 'hot cross bun' allows us to collect the information directly relating to the four key domains of CBT, and then explain this back to the patient to both check for understanding and accuracy.

| Activity 2.5 | *Critical thinking* |

Read again the case study on Richard, and then draw a 'hot cross bun' with his information.

An outline answer to this activity is provided at the end of the chapter.

As we have seen, explaining to your patient allows you to understand the nature of the problem, but it also allows your patient to understand what they might be doing that is likely to have an impact on their problem. For example, Richard might not have realised that when he ignored the call from his friends to go out that this might make him worse. Initially he could have felt relief, but later on he could have felt guilt at letting his friends down, which then links into his thoughts about being no fun, and the cycle starts all over again. Explaining this back to Richard is crucial to check that your understanding is correct, but it also allows Richard to gain some understanding of the impact that his behaviours have on his emotional state.

The 'hot cross bun' is a very simple 'formulation' or case conceptualisation. There are also specific formulation templates for specific problems that can aid the therapist in gathering the pertinent information and then displaying it in a way that allows the patient's problems to be understood in a more helpful format. There is not the space here to show every different formulation, and also the practitioner needs to be trained specifically in CBT to be able to use them fully, however the website 'Get Self Help' (**www.getselfhelp.co.uk/freedownloads.htm**) has examples of many of them.

Westbrook et al. (2011) describe the purpose of a formulation as being a description of the current problems, set against an account of how these problems might have developed with an understanding of the process that could be responsible for keeping the problems going. They describe the benefits of the formulation as being a better understanding of the problems by both therapist and patient and allowing what may be seen as a collection of random symptoms to be put together in a way that makes sense. They also provide a guide for the therapy that follows, because having a reasonable understanding of the problem allows the intervention to be specific to the patient and their problem, as opposed to a catch-all treatment that is generalised and not individual. The formulation also allows the patient to consider different explanations as to what is causing the problem, in an atmosphere of self-discovery as opposed to self-blame. It also allows the therapist and patient to predict potential difficulties in the therapy, or with the therapeutic process, and therefore how these might be avoided.

From this it becomes clear that it is not just the current problem that therapists need to consider, but also some of the process and behaviours that our patients may be doing to 'help' them to deal with it. I say 'help' as our patients have no wish to both prolong and intensify the problem and the things that they do are often done with the best intent; however, the action that happens can be counterproductive. It is therefore really important that we approach these behaviours with an open mind and a non-judgemental attitude. For example, in helping Richard, you may know that avoidance of social contact is a common feature of depression, but will not wish to tell Richard this. What can happen is that through the use of a formulation Richard is enabled to understand what he is doing that is maintaining the problem. These maintaining processes are very important, as they will be the factors that will keep the problem going, even when the original cause has disappeared.

Case study

Matilda, as a small child, was woken in the early hours of the morning by a spider crawling across her face. Since then she has avoided any rooms that are dusty or may contain spider's webs. In this case

> *Matilda's problem is maintained not by the original spider, which has long since perished, but the fact that she avoids anywhere where they may be spiders.*

Triggers and consequences

In Matilda's case it is not the spider that maintains her problem, it is the avoidance of any potential situation where there may be spiders, and this avoidance is a maintenance process, or safety behaviour. Safety behaviour neatly captures what it means for the patient, in Matilda's case the avoidance of spiders. It is therefore very important to gather information around the problem in the context of what the patient might be doing to improve the situation. An example of this might be a very direct question such as 'Is there anything that makes the problem worse, or better?'

We are now beginning to get a clearer picture of the problem from the patient's perspective, but we still need to gather further information to help us to really understand the full context of the problem, such as what triggers the situation and what are the consequences of the problem.

Triggers allow us to understand the situations where the problem is likely to occur. Triggers are important for two reasons: they give us clues as to possible beliefs or factors that may be maintaining the problem, and also they can be helpful to guide treatment. In Matilda's case the avoidance of many situations where she believes there may be spiders (the trigger) indicates that exposure to these situations to show her she can be safe is indicated as a treatment option. In Matilda's case the trigger is not necessarily a spider, it is any situation where Matilda feels that spiders may be present, for example dusty rooms or rooms with spider's webs. We must be careful not to assume what the trigger is and should both ask our patient and explore potential triggers to ensure that we understand these fully. We should also be aware that there might not be a trigger in terms of a specific situation, but it could be a thought or an image. An example of this in Matilda's case could be the thought of having to go up to get a box from the loft. In this case Matilda is not in the dusty environment, but is either having an image of it or is thinking about whether there will be spiders there.

Consequences allow us to gain a full perspective of the impact of the problem on the patient and therefore to understand what the patient has lost as a result of the problem. This is also an ideal opportunity to display some empathy towards the patient and recognise the efforts that the patient has made towards solving the problem themselves, both of which when acknowledged can aid in maintaining and establishing the therapeutic alliance.

Both triggers and consequences can be incorporated into our formulation, or 'hot cross bun', to complete the cycle. Triggers go above the 'hot cross bun' as a situational context and consequences below as a result of the symptoms. The use of a model such as Chris Williams's (2003) can help us to remember these and form a basis to relay our understanding back to our patients (see Figure 2.2).

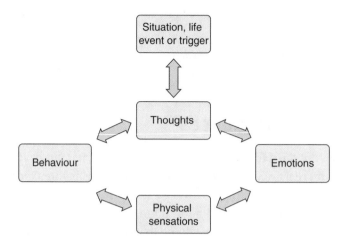

Figure 2.2: The five areas diagram used in CBT formulation

Understanding the assessment: validated and idiosyncratic measures

By now we should have a better and shared understanding of our patient's problem, which will allow us to begin to think about treatment. It is good to have an objective baseline measure of the impact of the problem so we can ascertain, in an objective and measurable way, whether treatment is leading to an improvement of the problem. This baseline measure can also serve to help us to put together a provisional diagnosis, along with all of our subjective information gained from the patient, and therefore be a guide as to what treatment should entail. This is described as a core competency for CBT therapists (Roth and Pilling, 2007). To do this we use what are commonly referred to as outcome measures. Outcome measures are reliable, validated and accurate tools that have been developed from research into specific conditions and symptoms (see Chapter 5). These tools are most commonly in the form of a series of questions that once completed allow a practitioner, or patient, to score their symptoms and measure them against values which we know, through research, are accurate against a profile of symptoms linked to specific conditions or diagnoses. There are literally hundreds of these measuring a range of conditions, so you need to use a measure that is specific to your patient's problem and will be useful for assessing the impact and quite possibly for measuring the success of treatment. A prime example of where this has been used to great effect is within IAPT. IAPT uses these measures not only to benefit the patient and practitioner, but also as a service evaluation tool, and as such can justify decisions around funding and allowing for targeting of specific groups of patients. We cannot here explore all possible ones which could be useful in a mental health setting but will consider a couple to help with the measurement of anxiety or depression within any context, e.g. primary care as well as secondary care.

Activity 2.6   *Reflection*

Think back to your last or current placement, where outcome measures could have been used. What did the staff use and why? Were the patients involved in either the administration of the outcome measure or the evaluation? Why might it be important to involve the patient in this process?

Both the Patient Health Questionnaire (PHQ 9; Kroenke et al., 2001) and the Generalised Anxiety Disorder assessment (GAD 7; Spitzer et al., 2006) are validated measures to measure depression and anxiety respectively, and are used in every patient therapy session within IAPT. The PHQ 9 is a nine-item questionnaire based around the diagnostic criteria for depression by the Diagnostic Statistical Manual (DSM) and gives a score that correlates to mild, moderate, moderately severe and severe symptoms of depression. The GAD 7 is a seven-item questionnaire measuring anxiety based on the DSM criteria for anxiety and giving a score that correlates to mild, moderate, moderately severe and severe symptoms of anxiety. As these are validated and reliable tools we know that a score of moderate anxiety is equivalent to moderate anxiety in a group of research subjects and is therefore clinically accurate. This, however, does not always mean that the scores match the presentation as sometimes patients can either under- or over-score for a number of different reasons. They should always therefore be used alongside a clinical assessment and should not be taken as indicative of depression or anxiety on their own. They then become a useful tool to help confirm a provisional diagnosis, but also to help monitor treatment from an objective perspective.

Activity 2.7 — *Evidence-based practice and research*

Using the reference at the end of the chapter obtain a copy of the PHQ 9 and or GAD 7 for you to complete. The aim here is not to see if you are depressed or anxious but to become familiar with the use of a tool such as this as understanding the barriers or difficulties of using such tools from a personal perspective will aid in your ability to use it with your patients (Bennett-Levy et al., 2001).

The scoring on these tools is relatively straightforward. For the PHQ 9:

5–10 representing mild symptoms;

10–15 moderate symptoms;

15–20 moderately severe;

20–27 severe.

The GAD 7 is also very similar,

0–5 mild symptoms;

5–10 moderate symptoms;

10–15 moderately severe;

15–21 severe.

These are just two of many tools that can be used to aid understanding, diagnosis and treatment, however there are a few points of caution to consider in using these and others. The tool needs to be either freely available for all clinical use, or have been purchased for use by the Trust before they can be used freely. Not doing this leaves you and your Trust open to litigation by the authors (the PHQ 9 and GAD 7 are both free to use). Some tools are designed to be administered by the clinician and some are self-report (such as PHQ 9 and GAD 7), and there are reasons as to why they are one or the other. The majority of Trusts now have psychologists employed to work in a variety of areas and they are valuable sources of advice and information around the use of any validated tool.

CBT does not however just rely on validated tools; it also uses subjective measures. These are important as they allow the therapist and patient to devise scorings and ratings that are individual to that patient. This is helpful as it allows the work to be customised to fit individual needs rather than trying to fit it into a validated tool. They are however idiosyncratic and as such can only be viewed in a subjective light but can be very useful to measure concepts such as belief in a thought or anxiety in a certain situation. These are often numerical in value and represent points on a continuum; for example when Matilda was asked to hold a jar containing a dead spider in an exposure session she reported her anxiety as being 95 out of 100. On its own, and without any explanation, this does not necessarily mean much, but when we understand that the therapist asked her to rate her current anxiety using a scale of 0 being no anxiety at all and 100 being the most anxious she had ever felt, it makes more sense. It is therefore very important to ensure that context behind both the use and meaning of the scale is established prior to using the measure. There are commonly used subjective measures such as anxiety or belief ratings, but there is no reason why a therapist could not design a subjective scale to fit a patient's presentation and clinical need. The caution to remember here is that this is not a validated tool, therefore the results cannot be generalised to other patients. For example we could not assume that because Matilda's anxiety around holding a dead spider in a jar was 95 out of 100 then most people would rate the same level of anxiety when holding a dead spider in a jar.

What does a CBT session look like?

Now we understand the type of information we need to gather and how we might measure it, but how do we put it all together?

CBT is by its nature structured in terms of the information gathered, and to do this it must also sit within a structure in terms of the session itself. We know that CBT is a collaborative project and therefore involves the patient as much as is possible in all aspects and requires active engagement both in and outside of therapy sessions. It is also problem focused and as such is generally time limited, although there are exceptions to this, particularly with the treatment of personality disorders and psychosis. However, these are for those trained in severe and enduring mental illness CBT and are out of the scope of this book.

When we considered the stepped approach used within IAPT services which uses two levels of CBT we can see that on average at Step 2 (a scaled down version of full CBT) a patient can expect

6–8 sessions of around 30–40 minutes, and on average at Step 3 (full CBT) a patient can expect 15–20 sessions of around one hour.

The first couple of sessions in full CBT are normally focused around both the assessment and formulation and checking this against the patient's experience. There is also what is often referred to as socialising the patient to the cognitive model, which is usual in both full and scaled down CBT, and involves educating the patient to the CBT model, most usually by use of the 'hot cross bun'. In addition there are a number of features, which are consistently used throughout the course of therapy, including the assessment stage:

- agenda setting;
- homework review;
- homework setting;
- reflection.

These features provide a base from which therapy can be consistently and coherently applied.

Agenda setting

Agenda setting serves a number of functions, primarily to be able to manage the time in the most efficient way possible. It also functions as an aid to collaboration where both therapist and client identify agenda items to be discussed within the session, and provides a regular feature to allow consistency across all sessions. A typical agenda will include items such as an update, a review of homework, a discussion around specific CBT techniques, items that the patient has identified as important to consider, setting homework and review of the session and course of therapy.

Homework

Homework, or work that is done outside of the session but based on things that are discussed within the session, is crucial to CBT. It allows the patient to be able to both contextualise and put into practice the learning that is established within the therapy session. Practically, it also allows for new information to be gathered and tested, which can then form the basis of a discussion in the following session. We have seen that CBT involves partnership working and the homework gives the patient an opportunity to 'own' the therapy personally. The majority of CBT therapists want their patients to become their own therapists and therefore being able to apply learning in a practical manner allows for the application of this learning to other examples. As an example, Matilda was treated with exposure therapy for her fear of spiders and now understands that anxiety will decrease in time. She can then apply this to other areas where anxiety causes her concern, for example at work when she has deadlines to meet. It also reflects the real world, as therapy sessions are often separate or isolated from real life. There is a great deal of evidence for the importance of homework, therefore it is essential that it forms part of the therapy process and therefore is given enough time within the session. This time needs to be divided between the review of homework and the setting of new homework. The review is important as it confirms the importance of the task to the patient, but also allows for new information or findings to be discussed in the context of the shared understanding of the patient's problems. Our patients do not always make the links, and we as therapists are there to help them attach this meaning and therefore to begin to apply it throughout their lives. Reviewing it also allows us to check if it has been completed, and therefore to identify any potential barriers. Remember when you were at school, there were teachers who always asked for the homework in, and those who did not always, and you soon realised which homework had to be completed on time! It may also be that the patient had 'life problems' which may have impacted on this, and therefore may be something that the therapist needs to assign some time to. It could also be that they did not understand the task and therefore assigning time to it allows for this to be fully resolved and plans to ensure that this does not happen again to be drawn up. The setting up of homework is therefore just as crucial and the following suggestions should help in ensuring that the homework is both relevant and is completed. It should follow on from what was discussed in session, and therefore be both logical and make sense to the patient. It is important to check out with the patient what they are capable of doing as our patients will have lives outside of therapy, and it is important that we do not give our patients too much to do as they are then likely to not complete it. Finally it is important that the homework is planned in significant detail; using 'what, where, when and with whom' can be useful in allowing this detail.

Reflection

Reflection is less of a specific item to be used in therapy, but is much more of a way of conducting therapy. It is important that both therapist and patient are able to reflect on what has happened to be able to find an adaptive and efficient way of solving the problem that the patient brought to therapy. This should underpin all of the work done in the session and as the patient learns how to use homework, or tasks outside of therapy, then this also forms a reflective element. To start with a reflection on the session itself can be useful, for example the therapist asking the patient what they have learnt today. This can be broadened out by the use of tools such as diaries to allow the patient to reflect on an experience, whether it is observational or a specific task undertaken. Reflection by the therapist on their own conduct of therapy is very important here as we must be aware that sometimes our own actions, be they verbal or non-verbal, can have an impact on our patients, and to be truly able to help them we must be aware of these to ensure that the most therapeutic environment is constructed for therapy with every patient. In terms of accessing this reflection we, as therapists, play this role in the therapy session, and we gain it through the use of supervision. It is also worth considering that the use of the techniques we ask our patients to use can greatly aid in this process, for example the use of a thought diary, or even a reflective account of a difficult situation. As supervision is crucial to unlocking this for us (and mirroring the process being observed within the therapy) it is vital that we have supervisors with whom we feel comfortable.

The use of technology

Before we move on to the interventions that we might use to move our patients into a treatment phase following the gathering of information and structures that we have established, it is important to consider the ways in which therapy can be delivered.

Traditionally CBT has been a face-to-face appointment of around an hour. This however does not always prove to be the most practical in terms of some of our patients who may lead busy lives and therefore the commitment of getting to an appointment, having the appointment and then getting back can take up to a few hours. We as therapists must therefore be open to 'moving with the times' and utilising modalities of contact, which suit the lives of our patients. IAPT has been a shining example in this context with the model developed around the use of the telephone (Richards and Whyte, 2011) as the medium of contact. The telephone however is not the only other modality and countries such as those in the Scandinavian bloc utilise email and internet delivery alongside the telephone. This also reflects the growing popularity of tools such as Skype generally speaking within our cultures, and as such should also be embraced as a tool to aid both engagement and accessibility of therapy to those to whom it seemed inaccessible. This is not to say that face-to-face does not have its place as it does; it just means that we should not discount alternative contact methods to be able to deliver therapy.

It is not just mediums of contact that we need to consider, but also multi-media as a whole. Conducting a search of the Apple app store recently revealed that there are a number of apps that are available to both help and support our patients with mental health problems. These can also be useful in our delivery, and could be as simple as using the note function on a phone to record thoughts, which save the potential embarrassment of writing it on a piece of paper at the time, or trying to remember it for later. A quick scan around any shopping centre will show many people on their phones, therefore will not be viewed by anyone with any curiosity. There are also apps, which provide more guided functionality in terms of anxiety and depression. Some caution should be exercised here as we are not advocating a specific app; in the nature of the iterative process of therapy we should encourage our patients to think of the resources that may assist them in the therapy and then reflect on how useful they are. There are no, to the author's knowledge, recommended apps by either the NHS or the Government for use in this area, and we cannot be seen as favouring one over another.

In the next chapter we consider what we can do to help our patients to develop more adaptive and positive ways to change their lives through the use of evidence-based CBT interventions.

Activities: brief outline answers

Activity 2.2 Reflection
Examining our own thoughts

Positive thoughts are on the whole very functional and therefore do not cause us any problems. This means that we would not necessarily wish to re-evaluate these.

Activity 2.3 Critical thinking
Identifying thoughts and behaviours

Cognitions (thoughts): 'I feel useless', 'I am no fun', 'no-one wants to spend time with me'.

Behaviours: staying in bed, not eating, ignoring the phone call, avoiding going out with his friends.

Activity 2.5 Critical thinking

What Richard's 'hot cross bun' might look like:

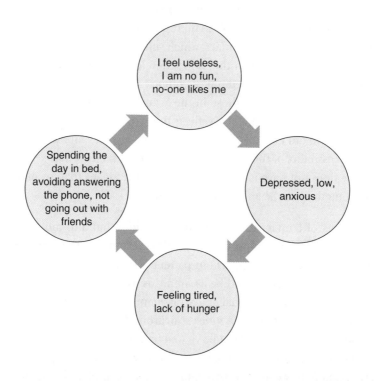

Further reading

Papworth, M, Marrinan, T and Martin, B (2013) *Low Intensity Cognitive Behavioural Therapy, a Practitioners Guide.* London: Sage.

Simmons, J and Griffiths, R (2014) *CBT for Beginners.* London: Sage.

Useful websites

www.getselfhelp.co.uk/freedownloads.htm
'Get Self Help' has examples of many useful tools to use in a CBT session.

www.moodgym.anu.edu.au
MoodGYM: Information, quizzes, games and skills training to help prevent depression.

www.livinglifetothefull.com
Living Life to the Full: Free online life skills course for people feeling distressed and their carers. Helps you understand why you feel as you do and make changes in your thinking, activities, sleep and relationships.

Chapter 3
Dialectical behavioural therapy: an introduction

Julie Roberts

NMC Standards for Pre-registration Nursing Education

This chapter will address the following competencies:

Domain 1: Professional values

All nurses must practise in a holistic, non-judgemental, caring and sensitive manner that avoids assumptions, supports social inclusion; recognises and respects individual choice; and acknowledges diversity. Where necessary, they must challenge inequality, discrimination and exclusion from access to care.

2.1 Mental health nurses must practise in a way that addresses the potential power imbalances between professionals and people experiencing mental health problems, including situations when compulsory measures are used, by helping people exercise their rights, upholding safeguards and ensuring minimal restrictions on their lives. They must have an in depth understanding of mental health legislation and how it relates to care and treatment of people with mental health problems

All nurses must work in partnership with service users, carers, groups, communities and organisations. They must manage risk, and promote health and wellbeing while aiming to empower choices that promote self-care and safety.

4.1 Mental health nurses must work with people in a way that values, respects and explores the meaning of their individual lived experiences of mental health problems, to provide person-centred and recovery-focused practice.

Mental health nurses must have and value an awareness of their own mental health and wellbeing. They must also engage in reflection and supervision to explore the emotional impact on self of working in mental health; how personal values, beliefs and emotions impact on practice, and how their own practice aligns with mental health legislation, policy and values-based frameworks.

Domain 2: Communication and interpersonal skills

All nurses must build partnerships and therapeutic relationships through safe, effective and non-discriminatory communication. They must take account of individual differences, capabilities and needs.

(continued)

continued ... ••

1.1 Mental health nurses must use skills of relationship-building and communication to engage with and support people distressed by hearing voices, experiencing distressing thoughts or experiencing other perceptual problems.

1.2 Mental health nurses must use skills and knowledge to facilitate therapeutic groups with people experiencing mental health problems and their families and carers.

2. All nurses must use a range of communication skills and technologies to support person-centred care and enhance quality and safety. They must ensure people receive all the information they need in a language and manner that allows them to make informed choices and share decision making. They must recognise when language interpretation or other communication support is needed and know how to obtain it.

3. All nurses must use the full range of communication methods, including verbal, non-verbal and written, to acquire, interpret and record their knowledge and understanding of people's needs. They must be aware of their own values and beliefs and the impact this may have on their communication with others. They must take account of the many different ways in which people communicate and how these may be influenced by ill health, disability and other factors, and be able to recognise and respond effectively when a person finds it hard to communicate.

All nurses must take every opportunity to encourage health-promoting behaviour through education, role modelling and effective communication.

6.1 Mental health nurses must foster helpful and enabling relationships with families, carers and other people important to the person experiencing mental health problems. They must use communication skills that enable psychosocial education, problem-solving and other interventions to help people cope and to safeguard those who are vulnerable.

NMC Essential Skills Clusters (ESCs)

This chapter will address the following ESCs:

Cluster: Care, compassion and communication

1. As partners in the care process, people can trust a newly registered graduate nurse to provide collaborative care based on the highest standards, knowledge and competence.

By the first progression point:

4. Shows respect for others.
5. Is able to engage with people and build caring relationships.

By the second progression point:

6. Forms appropriate and constructive professional relationships with families and other carers.

By entry to the register:

12. Recognises and acts to overcome barriers in developing effective relationships with service users and carers.

13. Initiates, maintains and closes professional relationships with service users and carers.

Chapter aims

By the end of the chapter, you should be able to:

- understand the components of a dialectical behavioural therapy (DBT) programme and their aims;
- suggest client groups for whom DBT may prove an effective treatment;
- describe the skills used in a DBT programme and how these may be used;
- practise DBT skills within you own daily life, realising how important it is that you believe in the skills when supporting a client to learn and practise them;
- discuss how to support a client undertaking a DBT programme.

Introduction

This chapter aims to provide you with a clear understanding of DBT, using the case studies of a real service user's journey through DBT. The chapter will explain the stages and skills incorporated within DBT and how you can support clients undergoing DBT. It will help you consider how you can use DBT skills in your own life. Not only will using the DBT skills help you, it will also show clients that you understand and believe in these skills, making it more likely they will want to learn them.

A little history

Dialectical behavioural therapy was developed by Marsha Linehan (1993b) originally to help women with severe borderline personality disorder (BPD) to reduce their self-harm and suicidal behaviour. This group can experience extreme emotions and it is often these, coupled with a tendency towards impulsivity, that leads to a pattern of destructive behaviour. The use of DBT is expanding to other groups (for example those with eating disorders (Palmer et al., 2003) and drug resistant depression (McKay et al., 2007) and in family therapy (Hoffman et al., 1999)). The skills outlined in this chapter can be useful for anyone experiencing strong emotions. If this is you, try them out and see! When you are helping clients to learn and practise these skills, it is a great motivator to them that you have tried them and believe in their ability to help.

Who can it help?

The main aim of DBT is to develop a life which is felt to be worth living by minimising behaviours that may presently been viewed as destructive, both in terms of a person's own health and of their functioning in society (e.g. forming relationships, maintaining employment). As clients start to build up a life that appears worthwhile this gives them a sense of mastery.

> ### Case study
>
> *At the commencement of DBT Millie thought that she would be 'cured' completely at the end of the programme and it came as a bit of a shock when she realised that she still has to work on regulating her emotions. 'I have come to see though that, pre-DBT, my illness largely controlled my life whereas now I am in charge, although I need to consider that there may be times when I need to work harder at regulating my emotions and perhaps slow down at times when things are slightly harder. This appears, to me, much like for someone with a chronic physical condition, e.g. asthma, diabetes'.*

In DBT the ideal view to be held by both clients and therapists is that:

- people in DBT are doing the best they can;
- people in DBT want to improve;
- people in DBT need to do better, to work harder and be motivated to change;
- the lives of suicidal individuals are unbearable as they are currently being lived;
- people in DBT must learn new behaviours in all areas of their lives;
- people cannot fail in DBT: if they are not progressing then it is viewed that the treatment itself is failing and that the therapist and client need to work upon which areas of the therapy need to change to assist progress.

Research summary: Studies of DBT and its effectiveness

DBT has demonstrated effectiveness in randomised clinical trials. In the first study conducted by Linehan et al. (1991) 47 chronically suicidal BPD patients were randomly assigned for a year either to DBT or to referral to treatment as usual in the community. During the year, DBT patients were less likely to attempt suicide or drop out (84 per cent remained in treatment). They spent much less time in psychiatric hospitals, had greater reductions in use of psychotropic medications and were better adjusted at the end of the year. They were also less angry than patients given standard psychotherapy (although at one year not less depressed or less likely to think about suicide). Most of these differences persisted a year after treatment ended.

It could be argued that DBT patients had a better outcome simply because they received more psychotherapy than the others. DBT though proved to be more effective even after researchers corrected for the amount of time spent with psychotherapists, and even after they excluded patients who received no individual psychotherapy. They are now conducting a large randomised clinical trial of DBT with a new group of therapists and patients.

A study conducted by Feigenbaum et al. (2012) looking specifically at outpatient DBT in community settings also demonstrated an improvement although suggested further studies are necessary to focus upon how the DBT process can be enhanced to improve effectiveness.

Dialectical behavioural therapy is mentioned in the National Institute for Health and Care Excellence (NICE, 2009) guidelines for the management of moderate to severe BPD.

The stages of dialectical behavioural therapy treatment

There are several distinct stages to DBT treatment.

Pre-treatment

This takes place usually over a 4–6-week period and aims to commence building the relationship with the therapist, establish the willingness of the client to undertake the treatment and to provide information on what the therapy will involve. The therapist signs a contract promising to deliver the treatment to the best of their ability and the client signs a contract promising to remain in therapy for the duration and to work on reducing self-harm and other behaviour which is having

Patient agreements	Therapist agreements
Stay in therapy for the specified time period	Make every reasonable effort to conduct competent and effective therapy
Attend scheduled therapy sessions	Obey standard ethical and professional guidelines
Work toward reducing suicidal behaviours as a goal of therapy	Participate in skills training for the specified period
Work on problems that arise that interfere with the progress of therapy	Be available to the patient for weekly therapy sessions and provide needed therapy back-up
	Maintain confidentiality
	Obtain consent when needed

Table 3.1: Commitments in dialectical behavior therapy

a significant impact upon their lives. There is usually a rule stating that if a client misses a certain number of skills or individual sessions then they are off the programme. This is usually strictly enforced. This is where the concept of dialectics sets in. Both client and therapist need to accept where the client is now, and the difficulties that s/he has presently and to acknowledge that these have occurred both through the client's actions and events that they have had no control over. They both need to acknowledge though that there is room for them to make changes in how they cope and regulate their emotions (see Table 3.1).

Stage 1 treatment (12 months)

The prominent aim of this stage is to reduce life-threatening behaviours and for clients to learn and practise a variety of skills. This aims to reduce the incidence of self-harm and the number of hospital admissions.

Stage 2 treatment (usually 6 months plus)

Many clients have experienced a variety of life traumas. This stage focuses on working on these post-traumatic stress responses. Stage 2 treatment can often not safely occur until the client has successfully completed Stage 1 treatment and has the skills to cope with the distressing emotions that discussing past events may trigger.

Stage 3 treatment (usually 6 months plus)

During this stage the client is supposed to move on to 'ordinary happiness and unhappiness' by dealing with problems of living.

There is even a *fourth stage*, which aims at an overcoming of a sense of incompleteness and the development of a 'capacity for sustained joy'.

In the UK individuals usually only undertake Stage 1 treatment, with some going on to work at Stage 2. This restriction may be because of lack of resources, or because the individual either does not wish or is not prepared to work on the other stages alone or that they move onto a different form of therapy after completing Stage 1. The initial stage usually takes place over a 12–18-month period and for the majority is community-based. In some instances it is carried out within a Therapeutic Community or inpatient setting.

Wind down stage (6 months)

After completing the skills training programme clients are usually given several further sessions with their individual therapist. This provides an opportunity for the client to adjust to the termination of the relationship and to discuss how they are going to move forward, or continue to develop their skills on completion of therapy and also identify the other sources of support that are available to them. Although the relationship is close between the therapist and client the fact that it is going to end at some stage is recognised right from the commencement of therapy and it should be actively discussed during the latter months of therapy. Many clients have experienced difficulties in establishing and maintaining relationships in their lives and describe the one with their therapist as the most successful and valued one they have ever had. Terminating the relationship, however much it is discussed, can be quite traumatic for the client and many take a while to adjust. It is hoped though that, as treatment has progressed, they have developed other sources of support, for example friends and family members in addition to professionals and also confidence in their ability to continue using the skills independently. Some areas have developed graduate skills groups where clients may be able to get together to discuss issues for several months after completing therapy.

The components of DBT

Skills training

This is usually carried out within a group setting. It is usually carried out weekly for between two and two-and-a-half hours. This is not group therapy and individual problems are not usually highlighted unless examples of how individuals are using specific skills are being discussed. There are usually ground rules set, for example not discussing self-harm within the group (as participants are trying to give this up and adopt more skilful methods of regulating their emotions!), confidentiality (what is discussed in the group stays in the room) and not forming exclusive relationships with other group members (which refers largely to clients being able to tell one of the facilitators if they are concerned about another).

Case study

The stance taken in Millie's group is that if a client chooses to ask either a fellow group member or therapist for support then they are expected to follow the advice given. She made friends with several members who had been in group alongside her. They were always careful to follow this rule. They did find the opportunity to discuss things with someone who had first-hand experience of what they were experiencing and the chance to bounce ideas off against each other was invaluable.

Skills groups can be quite nerve-wracking for some clients. Millie was extremely apprehensive about attending to begin with and also, at times, needed to contact her therapist afterwards as she was upset by how unwell some group members were. In some areas membership of the group remains static for the duration of the therapy. In the group Millie attended, clients commenced at the start of each module (see below). Having clients at varying stages of DBT treatment with differing levels of experience in using the skills often proves useful. Those in the early stages can be motivated and learn from those with more experience and those at a later stage of their treatment can potentially be inspired by how far they have come, gaining from assisting more junior members.

There is usually homework to complete between sessions where group members are expected to practise the skills learned before the next session. The initial part of a training session is devoted to encouraging the client to feed back on how they have found 'testing out' the skill and discussing any questions they may have surrounding this. If the client says they have not undertaken the homework they are asked to explain why and to discuss either how they could have used the skill or plan to do so over the next week. If this continues to occur then the individual therapist is informed and this is discussed during individual therapy sessions as it is viewed as a 'therapy-interfering' behaviour.

Millie said, 'I found I learned a huge amount from listening to how other clients had used the skills and was sometimes amazed by myself that I had used the skill which I only came to realise when providing homework feedback'.

Skills modules

There are four main groups of skills (often referred to as modules) covered, each being carried out over a 6–8-week period. These are distress tolerance, mindfulness, emotional regulation and interpersonal effectiveness.

In a full DBT programme each client usually undertakes each of these modules twice. In many areas this usually means repeating them a few months later. Millie said, 'I found I learned so much the first time round but found what I learned when repeating them (after I had gained more experience/practice) invaluable'.

Distress tolerance

This refers to a group of skills associated largely with helping clients 'get through' or cope with distressing events or circumstances. DBT is full of mnemonics. These can be quite confusing to both clients and staff initially, but when they have become more familiar they often help trigger ideas of additional strategies to try. There are a wide range of strategies designed to suit different situations and personal preferences.

Distraction with WISE mind 'Accepts' (see Mindfulness section)

A Activities: get involved in something (what would you choose to do?)

C Contributing: do something to help someone else out

C Comparisons: some may find it helpful to recognise their problems are similar or indeed not as dire as another person's; others may find it helpful to recognise changes in their own behaviour or responses (e.g. I would often have done this … but now I am …)

E Emotions: use opposite; if sad do something that may cheer you up, if lethargic do something to be active

P Pushing away: sometimes situations can be overwhelming; it may be appropriate not to think about them for a short period (not a long-term strategy but may provide time for an overwhelming emotional wave to pass)

T Thoughts: think of pleasant things

S Sensations: hot or cold items may help; some people splash cold water on the face; some use ice. Exercise also comes in this category

Self-soothe

Another technique is to use self-soothing, where you comfort yourself through stimulating the five senses (taste, smell, sight, hearing, touch). Clients are often encouraged to make a self-soothe box containing items for each of the senses so they are readily available for use when required.

Activity 3.1   *Reflection on action*

Plan and make your own self-soothe box. Place items in it that stimulate a variety of senses; try using it at times your feel stressed. Which sense do you find most powerful in helping?

There are outline answers and helpful ideas at the end of the chapter.

Here is another technique used in DBT to aid tolerance of distress.

'Improve' the moment

I Imagery: take your mind to a comforting safe place

M Meaning: try and see why something may be happening; it may possibly be that the meaning only becomes apparent at a later date

P Prayer: turning to a higher authority or being; this may or may not be religious

R Relaxation: e.g. progressively relax all the muscles in your body from head to toe

O One thing at a time: take things one thing at once

V Vacation: give yourself a break; may be to curl up on sofa or go somewhere; important that it is planned and time limited

E Encouragement: can come from both internal and external sources. Write a variety of encouraging statements (e.g. I can do this, I have got through situations like this before) and repeat these or write a list you can refer to

Pros and cons

In this strategy, you consider the pros and cons in relation to both doing or not doing something to help you reach a WISE decision. For example, it could be about whether to go out with friends or whether or not to engage in self-harming.

Activity 3.2   *Reflection in action*

Next time you have a decision to make and are unsure how to make it, try weighing up the pros and cons of both doing it and not doing it. Examples may include:

- whether to go to a party;
- whether to ask for help with an assignment;
- whether to discuss with your mentor an issue that is troubling your placement.

You may find, for example, that the pros of doing something are the same as the cons of not doing it, although you may identify other aspects that help you make a wise decision.

(continued)

continued ... •••

Use Table 3.2 to help. It may be that the WISE action (see mindfulness skills) comes from the longest list or it may be clear from reviewing what you have written which is the way forward. Writing things down may help you to stand back from the situation and consider things more clearly.

There are outline answers and helpful ideas at the end of the chapter.

Pros of doing	Cons of doing
Pros of not doing	Cons of not doing

Table 3.2: Pros and cons

Radical acceptance

This strategy means not struggling or fighting the current situation; you recognise it is as it is. You may not necessarily like it or agree with it, and it may not always be like this.

Willingness

This strategy involves being willing to do what is needed in each potential situation rather than being wilful, or not acting in the best interests of the situation even though this may be the way you want to act. This could be seen as 'cutting off your nose to spite your face'.

Some of these strategies are now illustrated by what happened to Suzy.

Case study

Suzy's boyfriend had called her last night to say that he wanted to finish the relationship as he had met someone else. Suzy, although initially very upset, now thought she had imagined the conversation, and that he was still deeply in love with her. She was still preparing for the night out at a party she had planned with him which he had told her would no longer be happening. She had not ACCEPTED what had happened and was still basing her actions on what she wanted. She was actually being incredibly WILFUL. She went to the party and he never showed up. She was angry and upset.

Next day she chatted to her friend who helped her recognise the facts of the situation. Suzy didn't have to like the situation and it may not always remain like this but at the moment Suzy needed to ACCEPT that this is how it is at this present time and be WILLING to work with it. Suzy agreed and threw her efforts into spending time with her friends. Her emotions became more manageable and her actions more effective.

Mindfulness

Mindfulness is a major strategy which aims to help you experience what is actually occurring in the present moment (see Chapter 4 for a more in-depth perspective). Often people get wrapped up with past problems and future fears and in so doing 'miss out' on what they can actually influence – the present moment. Observing the present also helps you stand back from what is happening and any thoughts and emotions associated with it and therefore helps you obtain what DBT refers to as WISE mind and plan a skilful way forward. Mindfulness also encourages you to be more compassionate towards yourself and to recognise and 'let go' of judgements (many of which are self-critical and serve to heighten emotions further).

Concept summary: States of mind in DBT

In DBT there are viewed to be three states of MIND which a person can largely be in (see Figure 3.1).

Emotion mind: when your thoughts, feelings and behaviour are largely controlled by your emotions. It is frequently described as hot, fiery and impulsive. Someone in this mind may be likely to hit out immediately if someone made them angry. It may be this impulsivity that leads to clients self-harming. It can, though, have benefits. It is often said that it is being largely in emotion mind that helps musicians and artists be most creative. It is the extreme love that enables a mother to get up, almost continuously, at night, to feed premature twins for several months!

Reasonable mind: when your thoughts, feelings and behaviour are largely controlled by fact and reason. For example, making a cake, when you mix ingredients by following instructions step by step. You may find yourself doing this in other areas of your life. Although at times it can be helpful it can make you feel quite detached from what you are doing as it does not consider your emotions. It may not therefore appear particu- larly relevant to you.

WISE mind: this is where both emotional and reasonable mind are considered to help you reach a balanced decision which takes account of both your emotions and the facts of the situation. It is seen as being greater than the sum of both put together as it adds a

(continued)

(continued)

further dimension. Therapists often show clients different coloured balls of play dough (one representing emotion mind and the other reasonable mind). Where they mix together there are a number of different colours, showing the richness of WISE mind.

Mindfulness is the vehicle for reaching WISE mind. Clients frequently ask how they know they have reached a WISE mind state, and it helps them to know that:

- often reaching WISE mind provides you with a sense of calmness; it often feels right; you may feel grounded;
- decisions reached in WISE mind often still appear the WISE way forward in a few hours' time; whereas those reached in the other two minds may change as, for example, your emotions change over time.

In the next activity, you can try analysing the different states of mind for yourself.

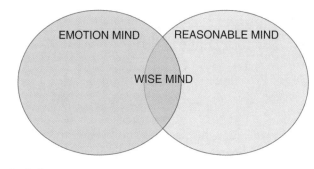

Figure 3.1: States of mind

Activity 3.3   *Critical thinking*

You are due to go out to a party. You are keen to impress everyone and have seen a really nice outfit you are desperate to have which costs £300. You cannot really afford it, though. You have a range of outfits at home that you have bought before and only worn once. You could wear one of those.

Consider the following:

- What may your EMOTION mind make you feel and want to do?
- What may your REASONABLE mind make you feel you should do?
- What would your WISE mind say? What may be the WISE course of action?

There are outline answers and helpful ideas at the end of the chapter.

Emotional regulation

When we regulate our emotions, we identify what we are feeling, and the precipitating factors for these feelings, and effectively manage these emotions without resorting to destructive behaviours.

These 'Please' behaviours can be used to help increase our tolerance of emotions. Used the wrong way, they can make us increasingly vulnerable to emotions.

P and **L** Treat **P**hysical **Il**lness

E Eating (sensible and balanced eating)

A Altering drugs (no drugs unless it is medication to be taken as prescribed by your doctor; includes alcohol and smoking!)

S Sleep (taking steps to assist in obtaining an appropriate amount, neither over nor under sleeping)

E Exercise

Activity 3.4 — *Reflection*

Think about times in your life when you may not have been properly attending to any of the items in the 'Please' list. For instance, you may have had a period of not having enough sleep. At such a time, was there a change in how you responded emotionally to events?

Consider whether you need to make any changes in your own life now, in relation to the 'Please' list. If so, make those changes and see how you feel in a week's time.

Mastery

Increasing a sense of mastery can assist in regulating emotions. Clients can plan or do something that increases their sense of control in either the short or long term. This sense of achievement can improve their mood and highlight to them their ability to control it.

Build positive experiences

One way of doing this is to create a list of things you have enjoyed or things that have gone well. Clients can make a bead jar and bank one bead for each experience alongside making a list of what they have achieved. When feeling down, looking at the jar or list often helps. Think about your own day. Can you identify one thing that has gone well?

Emotional experiences

Clients with BPD may experience difficulties identifying which emotion they are actually experiencing. The skills manual (Linehan, 2003a) contains lists of the signs and symptoms people may have when they experience the different emotions.

> ### Scenario
>
> *Millie reports finding it useful, at times, to draw a stickman, label what she is experiencing in different parts of her body and then to refer to these lists to assist identifying what emotion she is experiencing (see Figure 3.2). Imagine you are Millie's therapist: you could help Millie by considering an emotion as a set of physical symptoms and breaking them down into the individual symptoms and taking these one by one to make the emotion less overwhelming. You might relate this to having a cold. We may have a blocked nose, sore throat, headache etc. Considering these together can make us feel really unwell and sorry for ourselves. Thinking about each of these symptoms, one at a time, may help us to cope.*

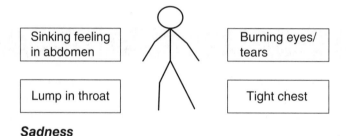

Sinking feeling in abdomen

Burning eyes/ tears

Lump in throat

Tight chest

Sadness

Figure 3.2: Millie's stickman

It is worth considering what triggered the emotion. Some clients feel at times emotions came from nowhere and arrived without warning (see Figure 3.3).

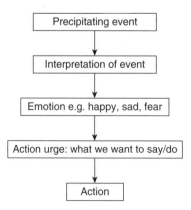

Precipitating event

Interpretation of event

Emotion e.g. happy, sad, fear

Action urge: what we want to say/do

Action

Figure 3.3: The emotional experience

Activity 3.5   *Reflection*

Take time to consider the action urges associated with each of the emotions in this table, and complete the table with examples of the actions urged.

Complete the following table.

Emotion	Action urge
Anger	Hit out, attack, shout
Sadness	
Joy/Happiness	
Guilt/Shame	

There are outline answers and helpful ideas at the end of the chapter.

Looking back at the table you completed in Activity 3.5, decide whether each emotion is warranted in a specific situation (and would be the same experienced by other people) or unwarranted (a different emotion to what others may experience) or unwarranted by degree (may be the same emotion experienced by others but either more or less intense).

If an emotion is warranted, then be mindful and sit with the current emotional wave as it passes; if happy then be happy, if feeling sad then cry if you need to.

If unwarranted or unwarranted by degree: act in a way opposite to the action urge associated with the emotion. For example, if the emotion is sadness do something active, if angry think kindly of yourself or another person.

Scenario

Emma is a therapist working with clients on DBT. When teaching she often describes the 'spider experience' as a way of explaining a warranted emotion.

If you are afraid of spiders and see a spider in the outback of Australia (which potentially could be poisonous) then your fear may be WARRANTED: it may cause you some harm.

If you see a spider in the UK (unlikely to be poisonous) and you responded with the same degree of fear you could say that your fear may be UNWARRANTED BY DEGREE.

If you see a dark blob that you think is probably dust (but may just be a spider) then if you respond with the same degree of fear as above then your fear may be UNWARRANTED.

Imagine you are explaining this to clients. What example would you choose?

Activity 3.6   *Decision making*

Consider how you may 'act opposite' to the emotion you are experiencing.

By acting opposite we are acting in a way completely opposite to the action urge associated with the emotion.

Complete the following table – you may like to refer back to Activity 3.5 to consider the action urge associated with the emotion.

Emotion	How to 'act opposite' to the action urge
Anger	Be kind to yourself; be or think kindly of the other person
Sadness	
Joy/Happiness	
Guilt/Shame	

There are outline answers and helpful ideas at the end of the chapter.

Case study

Amy's son, James, had recently started secondary school. Although his friends were taking packed lunches he wanted money to buy school lunch. Although Amy felt she should encourage him to do the same as his friends, she agreed. James returned from school upset and hungry. He had stayed with his friends, had no lunch and blamed Amy. Amy felt very guilty, apologised profusely to James, became hysterical and ended up rowing with a friend over the phone.

Later she considered the events and thought about what she would say to a friend in a similar situation. She had agreed to do what James wanted as she felt he was old enough to decide himself and it was only the fact no one else went to the canteen that had led to the subsequent events. From a DBT perspective her guilt was probably UNWARRANTED. She needed to ACT OPPOSITE to this guilt rather than being completely consumed by it and not let it drive her behaviour. Making James a large tea and discussing what to do the next day with him would have been more skilful.

- *Do you feel Amy's shame was warranted? Was she to blame for what happened to her son that day?*
- *What would you say to Amy if she described the situation to you?*

Interpersonal effectiveness

This set of DBT skills assists people in asking for what they want or being able to say no, but to balance these with the important facets of maintaining good relationships and self-respect.

These can be considered as a triangle (see Figure 3.4). Each is important although in some instances one may take precedence.

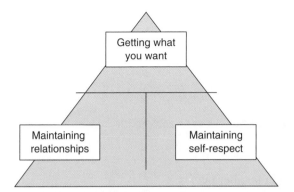

Figure 3.4: The goals during an interpersonal interaction

Let us look now at some mnemonics of skills which help with interpersonal effectiveness.

'Getting what you want/need/deserve'

('Dear man' skills)

D Describe what you want

E Express how you feel

A Assert what you want clearly

R Reinforce how it will benefit the other person

M Mindful focus on the situation as it is

A Appear confident

N Negotiate: be prepared to negotiate

Activity 3.7   *Communication*

Consider a situation during which you either have needed to or are going to need to ask for something you want or need. Rehearse what you may say using the structure above. This could either be a verbal conversation or the same skills can be effective in a letter or email. Ensure you ask clearly for what you want/need (as it may be that the person cannot second guess this) and that when you reach the reinforce part what may act as a reinforcement to them.

Try the situation and then consider how you have found it.

Although 'Dear man' skills are helpful, remember that in life we cannot always get what we need or want. This does not mean that we have not asked effectively: there are numerous factors involved in any situation. We only make up 50 per cent of any interpersonal interaction.

Maintaining a relationship

('Give' skills)

G Gentle approach

I Interested

V Validate

E Easy manner

Maintaining self-respect

('Fast' skills)

F be Fair to yourself and the other person

A do not be overly Apologetic

S Stick to your values

T be Truthful

Telephone coaching

In DBT, clients are encouraged to contact (usually) their individual therapist via text or pager if they need assistance. The aim of this is to encourage and/or coach them in learning to use the skills in dealing with issues as they arise in their daily lives. Although they may access regular support mechanisms, gaining coaching from the person who perhaps knows them best and is aware which DBT skills they are presently working on is invaluable. The telephone calls are usually short (5–10 minutes) as they are not aimed at being therapy sessions but aim to help deal with a specific issue as it arises. It can then be discussed further, if necessary, during the individual therapy session.

For many clients this often progresses, as therapy continues, from the individual initially recognising when they need help, to helping them to select and apply a skill, to then perhaps discussing other approaches to use if the initial one selected was not proving very effective.

It is up to the individual therapist to decide the times s/he is available for contact. As the therapist will not always be able to 'get back to' the client immediately, the client should have a plan B as to who to contact. Many therapists worry that they will be called on at very frequent intervals and put under high pressure by highly suicidal clients. Many therapists say this is rarely the case and clients are usually highly respectful of this coaching. As Dunkley (2012) says, if it was too onerous a task, therapists would not be prepared to do it and it would not form part of the treatment. If they are contacted too frequently or at inappropriate times then this is viewed as 'therapy interfering behaviour' and would be reviewed during an individual session. If a therapist is concerned about a client's safety then they will also be aware of and able to access the CRISIS response services within their Trust. Little (2009) states that even a highly suicidal client can often be talked around and encouraged. It is often comforting to the client when it is pointed out that the fact that they have asked for help proves they are being skilful and want to continue living. There is often a rule that if a client has engaged in any self-harm/suicidal activity then s/he is unable to contact the therapist for 24 hours following this (unless they need help in obtaining emergency treatment).

> ## Case study
>
> *Millie's therapist stated that coaching is a method of asking for help in using the skills to regulate emotions effectively without resorting to destructive behaviour. If Millie has chosen to harm then she no longer required the support to use skilful behaviour as she has 'already chosen her action'. In such a case, she was to text '24 hour rule' to her. Although there were other factors involved the fact of having to do this acted as a deterrent to self-harming. Millie found this aspect of the therapy the most useful and really appreciated her therapist who spent time coaching during evenings and weekends. Discussing and practising a skill in the classroom environment when you are frequently calm is very different from practising it alone in a highly charged emotional situation. It was then that Millie needed help, and she learned the most when supported in practising the skill within this arena. After completing DBT if Millie is struggling she texts herself as she would have texted her therapist during DBT. Reading the text enables her to 'stand back' from the situation and consider what advice she would give to a friend in the same situation. This has helped Millie act skilfully on a number of occasions.*

The more skilful you are the more support ...

Testing out the new skills and learning to regulate emotions skilfully can be hard work and very draining. Some clients have explained that they are sometimes reluctant to admit they are applying the skills and that they are helping for fear that support may be withdrawn or therapy finished early when indeed they are still finding things tough and need the support. DBT recognises this and frequently adopts the ethos that 'the better you do the more you get'. When the client is demonstrating that they are using the skills and working hard the therapist is motivated into helping more and providing more support. The client clearly recognises that by asking for help skilfully, rather than resorting to self-harm, more rather than less support is provided. Millie's therapist was always pleased for her to contact her when she had used a skill successfully and provided her with the same time as when she skilfully asked for help. This is a valuable lesson to learn for assisting clients to learn the skills necessary to form and maintain interpersonal relationships with others (which, as Linehan, 1993b and Linehan and Dimeff, 2001 state, some clients with BPD may experience difficulties with).

Although not paramount within the literature Millie's therapist and Millie viewed their partnership as being like a detective agency. They discussed a particular issue and how it may most effectively be handled or most closely identified. Millie then went and tested it out before returning to discuss her findings. They were then able to adapt strategies as necessary.

Group consultation

This part does not include the clients. DBT is a team treatment. The therapists (who may be psychologists or other mental health professionals who have undertaken DBT training) meet with each other usually once a week. The aim is to discuss issues arising within skills training, support each other and discuss the most effective method of dealing with issues arising for individual clients. Client progress can be slow in DBT. Consultation meetings are important in encouraging and motivating therapists to continue working with clients and perhaps assist them in identifying progress. It can obviously be highly stressful working alongside a group of highly suicidal clients; therefore working as part of a team and being able to draw on the support, experience and suggestions made by other professionals is paramount.

Relationship between the therapist and client

This is central to the concept of DBT. It is often one of the significant factors that motivates the client to remain in therapy and at times may be the one that keeps the client alive during difficult periods. The client is being encouraged to 'give up' destructive methods of coping which they may have been using for years, having found them helpful in assisting them to deal with extreme emotions and to replace these with a set of skills. During DBT you are asking the client to 'give up' unskilful behaviours whilst they are still learning and have not practised at length or perhaps fully 'tested out' that these skills can be effective. Millie found the initial few months of DBT hard. She felt she had entered into the programme with a significant number of problems but after starting to work alongside her therapist she felt she had a lot more. Millie found this frightening and demoralising and if it had not been for the constant encouragement and confidence of her therapist she feels she would have given up.

There has been much research undertaken on the importance of the therapeutic relationship during DBT. Linehan (1993a,b) acknowledges the relationship as central to the success of DBT and one of the differentiating factors between this and other therapy modes. Swales and Heard (2007) explain the aim being to create a collaborative relationship in which a warm and facilitative environment encourages the new learning and practice of skills to occur. The therapist role is often viewed as acting as a consultant to the client. Instead of 'solving problems' for the client the therapist provides the guidance and encouragement so the client can perform the actions themselves. If, for example, the client is experiencing difficulties working alongside another professional then, instead of 'taking over' and speaking to the professional themselves, the therapist coaches the client with regards to communicating most effectively.

Individual therapy

The therapist and client meet on a weekly basis usually for 45–60 minutes. Throughout the week the client completes a diary card daily including factors such as:

- suicidal urges/ideation (usually on a scale of 0–5 and any episodes of self-harm);
- intensity of emotions experienced;
- skills used and the ease with which the client feels they have used these.

The card is reviewed at the start of each therapy session. If not completed then the therapist may ask the client to complete one then.

The session focus is then decided and is based upon the following hierarchy:

- if any suicidal behaviours/self-harm has occurred this forms the basis of discussion;
- if suicidal ideation/urges are high;
- any therapy interfering behaviours (e.g. disruptive behaviour or not engaging in skills group, inappropriate use of telephone contact, not completing homework, being late or not attending a session);
- if none of these are present then the therapist and client can select what to focus upon. This may be an ongoing issue or one that has proved particularly pertinent in the past week. Millie's therapist frequently allowed her to select what they discussed. The opportunity to do this and to discuss areas she was finding particularly challenging acted as a strong motivator not to have engaged in the previous behaviours as otherwise these would have to form the priority.

During the sessions chain analyses are completed. A chain analysis is a technique designed to help a person understand the function of a particular behaviour. During a chain analysis of a particular problem behaviour (for example self-harm) the aim is to uncover all the factors that led up to that behaviour. In other words, a person tries to discover all the links in the chain that ultimately resulted in a problem behaviour.

Starting from the prompting event a person may identify the situation s/he was in, the thoughts s/he was experiencing, or the feelings s/he was having just prior to engaging in that behaviour. In doing so, a person can increase his/her awareness of all the factors that may put him/her at risk of a problem behaviour and during the behaviour itself. The last part involves identifying the consequences of the behaviour including how it made him/her feel. The client can then hopefully identify skills/actions that they could have taken to help direct behaviour in a different direction. It can also be used to help identify times that skilful behaviour has taken place.

In the early stages of DBT the therapist and client may complete these together but as therapy progresses clients are often encouraged to initially complete these themselves and to take these to discuss with their therapist.

As the example in Figure 3.5 shows, it is possible to show a chain/pathway between the precipitating event and consequent behaviour. As Millie progressed through DBT she was able to recognise linkages and that emotions and behaviour do not appear from nowhere. As she was able to do this she came to recognise that she did have a choice with regards to how she acted in response to events and the type of events that were most likely to lead her to behaving unskilfully. Millie was then able to observe how, using a variety of DBT skills, she could play a role in regulating emotions/coping with distress/managing behaviour at various stages. As she began to do this she was able to utilise skills at an earlier stage and prevent things from progressing. She also recognised and became more skilled at pausing after an event/emotion/thought prior to acting. This frequently enables 'WISE MIND' to take effect and ensure more skilful behaviour. Others have said it helps them to appreciate that even if a potentially self-harming behaviour (e.g. drinking excessively, cutting yourself) provides short-term immediate relief there are often longer term consequences that may not be so desirable.

Crashed car into wall at work and scratched paint work

⬇

Felt wave of panic and anger at myself

⬇

Thoughts of: 'what is my husband going to say?'

'How am I going to afford to get it fixed?'

'How am I going to get to work with no car?'

⬇

Anger at self increased

⬇

Thoughts/judgements:

'I am always doing stupid things'

'I lost my phone last week'

'I should have been more careful'

'If I bumped into a person instead of the wall I

could have really hurt them'

'There's something seriously wrong with me'

⬇

Went home

Consumed large quantity of alcohol

Initially felt a lot better

⬇

Overslept next morning and woke feeling hungover

⬇

Phoned in sick to work; felt very guilty

Using DBT skills

Anger: probably warranted to a degree; need to notice it, be mindful of it as a wave rising and falling and then let it go

Panic/fear: possibly unwarranted; nobody had been hurt. Act opposite by making decisions re practical tasks

Mindful of thoughts: notice them and 'let them go'; use guided imagery if necessary

---

Unwarranted by degree: act opposite by possibly showing kindness to yourself; think of some things you have done well or someone else says you have done well

Mindfulness of judgements

Was this really most skilfull behaviour? Show kindness to yourself e.g. self-soothe skills, take any practical steps to arrange repainting car

Figure 3.5: Example of chain analysis

Case study: Before and after

Pre undertaking DBT

Donna's son, Sam, came home from school yet again in tears. He'd been laughed at again and kicked by the same gang as upset him yesterday. He's only 6. They have no right to do this. Donna feels tense and then has the urge to hit out or grab the phone and complain to school. STOP! 'I have no right. He's been hurt enough. It's all my fault. I didn't bring him up properly. If only I'd gone out of my way to go to more parent and toddler groups he would have been able to socialise better'. Tears welled up in Donna's eyes. She had a hollow pain in her chest and her throat felt tight. She swallowed them down and put on a brave smile. 'I mustn't cry in front of him – I've failed him enough already'. She reached out to him and cuddled him. Donna didn't feel close to him – there was a barrier between them. Her face turned red, her muscles tightened. She needed to hide. 'I had caused this for him and now couldn't even comfort him! What sort of mother am I!'

Donna rapidly charged around the house busying herself. 'I must not get upset. I must not get upset. I must prove to everyone I am a good mother. Even my house is untidy. This just about sums it up doesn't

it! Why is this happening? Every aspect of my life is going wrong. My physical health, my marriage, my other kids are going to suffer the same fate – I haven't made any friends for them either'. The lump in her throat grew and her heart pounded faster.

'I've no right to be upset. I've caused it. It's because I've been ill. I was bullied at school so they've inherited it from me. Can't tell my husband – he'll blame me'. Donna's face becomes red, her heart rate increases, there's a sinking sensation in her chest. 'I want to run. Don't know what I feel – just know it's awful and I can't stand it'. Suddenly she feels numb. 'I'm floating. I have no right to feel like this. My feeling is scaring me. I'm confused'. A sense of panic and terror rises. 'I'm going to explode. I've got to escape. I've got to get out. I need to break this cycle'. She waits for her husband to get home. 'I no longer need to carry on. I can escape'. Donna reaches up for the pills at the top of the cupboard.

1 week ago (some time after completing DBT)

Sam came home from football training. The same boy had made nasty comments about him and tripped him up. There is a large gash on his leg. Donna feels tense and has the urge to run to the coach and complain. The anger quickly turns to sadness – why has this happened to him? What has he done to deserve it? Tears well up in her eyes, pain in the pit of her stomach, her heart rate increases, there's a lump in her throat. 'Definitely sadness, certainly warranted – any mum would feel this and yes I don't think I'm catastrophising so my level of sadness is warranted so need to be mindful and act with it'. Donna reaches out to Sam and cuddles him. Tears stream down his face and Donna sheds a few WILLING tears. She feels close to him and doesn't push him away. Ten minutes later they both feel better and go and raid the chocolate cupboard. (Think they deserved to self-soothe!) Twenty minutes later he is in the bath and the two of them are having a bubble fight – 'I'm being completely mindful as is he!'

*After he's in bed Donna starts thinking – 'Why is this happening to him, it must be my fault, I've been unwell, I'm a bad mother'. Her heart rate increases, her sense of panic rises, she feels breathless, then starts to feel floaty and numb. She can't quite think straight. Donna senses it is time to take action. She stops, sits down and grounds herself being aware of how her body contacts the chair and floor. Donna concentrates on physiologically calming herself (cold water followed by progressive muscle relaxation). Things slot back into perspective. She decides to keep an eye on the situation and speak to the coach if it reoccurs. 'This feels right – **wise** I suppose!'*

Donna wants to share how she is feeling. She reaches for the telephone and rings her friend Sarah. Donna explains things to her. She sympathises, kids eh! They joke and plan to meet for coffee the next day. They end up giggling over a television programme. She puts the telephone down. She read a chapter of her book and falls asleep when her head hits the pillow!

How nurses and other professionals assist clients undertaking DBT

DBT can appear complex, perhaps exaggerated by the many mnemonics that are included within it. This has often led nurses to say they don't understand DBT and telling clients to go to their therapists for help or simply to 'use their skills'. However, there are several ways that nurses can help.

Be aware of the hard work and effort that it takes to undertake a DBT programme (Lynch and Robins, 1997) and to provide general support, understanding and encouragement with regards to this.

Become familiar with a few DBT skills and terminology and mnemonics.

Validate what clients say; not merely saying 'things will get better' but showing that you understand that what they are going through is going to be particularly tough for them and this makes sense within their situation (Lynch and Robins, 1997 explain this well).

Show an interest if clients want to discuss how they are using their skills to manage a difficulty.

DBT encourages clients to ask for help clearly rather than using other attention-seeking behaviours. Listen to this; a client who is able to verbally comprehend and express their problem and that they need help may be in as much need and distress as one who cries or screams.

If unsure how DBT may approach a situation, then be truthful and explain this to the client and point them in the direction of someone with more knowledge.

Recognise how difficult the client may find finishing DBT and be aware they may, at least initially, require more support and understanding at this time.

Chapter summary

To conclude DBT is becoming an increasingly popular and widespread form of treatment for clients meeting the diagnostic criteria for BPD although its use is spreading to clients experiencing other difficulties. This chapter has aimed to provide readers with an insight into the DBT process both in terms of what it includes in addition to what Millie learned through her own personal DBT journey. The chapter has also aimed to enable students to consider how they can play a role in caring for clients undergoing DBT even if they are not personally involved with the provision of DBT and to facilitate them in experiencing using DBT skills within their own personal life.

Activities: brief outline answers

Activity 3.1 Reflection on action

Self-soothe box. Suggested items may be Touch: fabric, teddy bear, rock, hand cream; Vision: pictures, photographs, lava lamp; Hearing: CD; Taste: chocolate, favourite food; Smell: perfume, incense sticks.

Activity 3.2 Reflection in action

Going to a party:

Pros of going	Cons of going
Will enjoy it, all my friends are going, I have accepted invite already	I'm too tired, afraid I may meet Simon
Pros of not going	**Cons of not going**
Can go to bed early, won't have to meet Simon	Will feel guilty as will let my friend down, may actually have enjoyed it

Activity 3.3 Critical thinking

Emotional mind: really like it, would stand out in front of others. Action: buy on impulse.

Reasonable mind: cannot afford it, have other things that I need to buy. Price may reduce during a sale. Action: do not buy it, wait.

Wise mind: really like it but would probably only wear it once, I have other clothes I could wear at home. Action: consider what I have at home, perhaps buy accessory to go with existing dress.

Activity 3.5 Reflection

Emotion	Action urge
Anger	Hit out, attack, shout
Sadness	Cry, withdraw, seek comfort from others or soothe yourself
Joy/Happiness	Smile, socialise, sing, do more of the thing that has made you happy
Guilt/Shame	Hide away, avoid person, punish yourself

Activity 3.6 Decision making

Complete the following table – you may like to refer back to the previous exercise to consider the action urge associated with the emotion.

Emotion	How to 'act opposite' to the action urge
Anger	Be kind to yourself; be or think kindly of the other person
Sadness	Do something to cheer yourself up Make contact with someone
Joy/Happiness	Decide what may be warranted emotion and act accordingly
Guilt/Shame	Make a repair (say sorry), learn from the experience

Further reading

The following titles are useful both for clients undertaking DBT and also for professionals who are learning about DBT and supporting clients in learning and practising the skills. They all include case studies and practical examples directly relevant to the clinical areas in which students will encounter this client group.

Gratz, K and Chapman, AL (2009) *Freedom from Self-Harm: Overcoming self-injury with skills from DBT and other treatments.* Canada: New Harbinger.

Pederson, L and Pederson, LS (2012) *The Expanded Dialectical Behavior Therapy Skills Training Manual: Practical DBT for self-help, and individual and group treatment settings.* USA: Premier Publishing.

Swales, MA and Heard, HL (2009) *Dialectical Behavioural Therapy Distinctive Features.* East Sussex: Routledge.

Useful websites

www.dbtselfhelp.com

www.get.gg/dbt.htm

These websites are designed to support clients in practising DBT skills. They include examples of how people have used the skills in everyday situations and also discuss some of the challenges that clients may experience when using them. They are useful sites to direct clients to.

Chapter 4
Mindfulness for all in action

Julie Roberts

NMC Standards for Pre-registration Nursing Education

This chapter will address the following competencies:

Domain 1: Professional values

4.1   Mental health nurses must work with people in a way that values, respects and explores the meaning of their individual lived experiences of mental health problems, to provide person-centred and recovery-focused practice.

8.1   Mental health nurses must have and value an awareness of their own mental health and wellbeing. They must also engage in reflection and supervision to explore the emotional impact on self of working in mental health; how personal values, beliefs and emotions impact on practice, and how their own practice aligns with mental health legislation, policy and values-based frameworks.

Domain 2: Communication and interpersonal skills

All nurses must build partnerships and therapeutic relationships through safe, effective and non-discriminatory communication. They must take account of individual differences, capabilities and needs.

1.1   Mental health nurses must use skills of relationship-building and communication to engage with and support people distressed by hearing voices, experiencing distressing thoughts or experiencing other perceptual problems.

1.2   Mental health nurses must use skills and knowledge to facilitate therapeutic groups with people experiencing mental health problems and their families and carers.

All nurses must take every opportunity to encourage health-promoting behaviour through education, role modelling and effective communication.

Domain 3: Nursing practice and decision-making

8.1   Mental health nurses must practise in a way that promotes the self-determination and expertise of people with mental health problems, using a range of approaches and tools that aid wellness and recovery and enable self-care and self-management.

....

NMC Essential Skills Clusters (ESCs)

This chapter will address the following ESCs:

Cluster: Care, compassion and communication

1. As partners in the care process, people can trust a newly registered graduate nurse to provide collaborative care based on the highest standards, knowledge and competence.
6. People can trust the newly registered graduate nurse to engage therapeutically and actively listen to their needs and concerns, responding using skills that are helpful, providing information that is clear, accurate, meaningful and free from jargon.
....

Chapter aims

By the end of the chapter, you should be able to:

- explain the concept of mindfulness and the benefits that it may have for people practising the technique;
- discuss which client groups it may be useful for;
- describe how to perform an activity or exercise mindfully;
- evaluate a variety of different mindfulness exercises from experience;
- discuss the difficulties people may experience when learning mindfulness and how these may be overcome;
- discuss the role of the nurse in working alongside clients learning and practising mindfulness techniques.

Introduction

Do you ever feel totally engulfed by what is happening in your life? Events can throw us off balance and challenge our ability to cope. Mindfulness is a technique used at times like these. This chapter aims to introduce you to the concept of mindfulness, how it is presently being used and how and why it may be useful for yourself and your clients. There are examples of a range of mindfulness exercises, to enable you to practise and to reflect upon how you have found the experience. It also includes suggestions on how you can support someone learning mindfulness. All the activities are individual practices so there are no outline answers provided.

The first case study shows it is often not the event itself that throws us off balance, but our thoughts, interpretations, judgements, emotions and consequent actions. Williams and Penman (2011) suggest that a few sad thoughts can trigger a cascade of unhappy memories and lead to us feeling swamped.

Case study

Jodie was driving home from work. Although concentrating on the road, her mind was still thinking over the meeting she had attended. She was late home and knew it was going to be a rush to get ready to go out again. A car seemed to appear out of nowhere. Jodie tried to avoid it but it crashed into the front of her and forced her to the side of the road. No-one was hurt but Jodie realised her car was un-drivable. The other driver was not overly apologetic although he exchanged insurance details before driving off. Jodie, although initially calm, felt herself growing angrier and angrier. 'I just saw red and the next moment was in the midst of a full scale argument with the other driver'. How was she going to get home? Why hadn't the other driver looked where he was going? Had she really been paying attention? Her mind then switched to considering the inconvenience of having no car over the next few days and also to a colleague she had disagreed with at the meeting. She felt her anger building and building.

You can see how Jodie's anger grew as she considered other things that had made her angry in the past, and events that may make her feel this way in the future, compounded by the judgements she had about herself and others on these issues. As Williams and Penman (2011) suggest it is this cascade that can make us feel anxious, stressed and exhausted, which in some people can be prolonged and lead to serious clinical depression.

We may feel we have little control. As Jodie stated 'I just saw red and the next moment I was in the midst of a full scale argument'. Although Jodie may have been unable to prevent the accident, she does have control over how she responds to it. Although we cannot always change the present (the accident has happened and needs dealing with) we do have control over how we deal with it in this present moment. Do we hit out in anger or work through it, however much we may not like it? Although in many cases the actions may not be catastrophic, for a person with borderline personality disorder (BPD) this torrent of extreme emotions and potential impulsivity may precede self-harm and suicide attempts and may affect their interpersonal relationships with others.

Do you ever feel you are rushing so quickly through your life you are not really living in it?

Case study

Kate juggles a full-time job, running a house and caring for her son and daughter. She rushes from work to collect them from school prior to starting a run back and forwards to after-school clubs. Then there is dinner to cook, the house to clean and work for the next day to prepare for. As Kate is exhausted and really wanting to climb into bed her husband returns from work demanding her time and attention. Kate often tries to multi-task and frequently works in the car whilst waiting for the kids. She realises she doesn't really enjoy her life, didn't even see her son score a try during rugby as her mind was elsewhere and is always trying to 'move onto the next thing'. She notices she is becoming increasingly stressed, irritable and despite being exhausted can't sleep. She can't understand why as to her she has everything – kids, job, husband, friends and a nice house.

Kate is so preoccupied with juggling the many facets of her life that she is always rushing forward to the next event and not 'living' the present. She recognises her children are growing up quickly and she is not fully experiencing the pleasure of their achievements. Life is passing her by. Her general practitioner advised her to try and pace herself. When she slowed down she became more aware, enjoyed the pleasurable times and actually found she achieved more.

What is mindfulness?

Kabat-Zinn (2003) describes mindfulness as the ability to be aware of your thoughts, emotions, physical sensations and actions without judging yourself or your experience.

> *Mindfulness is the awareness that emerges through paying attention on purpose, in the present moment, and non-judgementally to the unfolding of experience moment by moment.*
> (Kabat-Zinn, 2003)

As Linehan (1993b) and Rezek (2012) explain, it is a conscious action that requires us to choose to be alert and pay attention on purpose to what is happening at this present moment in time. Through this we learn to live in the present moment rather than brooding about the past or worrying about the future. Linehan (1993b) stresses that participating without awareness (mindlessly) is often characteristic of impulsive behaviours.

The case studies epitomise the need to be mindful. Both Jodie and Kate could help themselves by living in the present rather than being heavily influenced by the past or future. In this way we may be able to reduce worry and stress, tolerate difficult times without feeling completely overwhelmed, gain greater control of our lives and actions and in many cases experience greater fulfilment.

Activity 4.1 — *Reflection*

How often is your body in one place and your mind in another? Do you recognise any of the following?

- Arriving at a place but not remembering how you actually got there?
- Having a conversation with someone but not really focusing upon what they are saying as your thoughts are elsewhere?
- Reading a page of a book and then having no recollection of what you read?

Yesterday is history, tomorrow is mystery. Today is a gift which is why it is called the present.
(The Dalai Lama)

Through developing greater awareness of present events we are able to step back slightly and be more in control of our mind and actions rather than letting our mind control us. When used in dialectical behavioural therapy (DBT), mindfulness encourages the client to stop before acting impulsively, balance emotional and rational minds (see Chapter 3) and find 'WISE MIND' before moving forward. This greater sense of personal control or influence was found by Kabat-Zinn (1979) when he first developed mindfulness for use with patients suffering from chronic pain. Speca et al. (2000) and Witek-Janusek et al. (2008) recognised a similar finding in those experiencing cancer. It helps many to recognise that they can shift their lives into a more manageable state and have greater control over their daily lives rather than letting the disease process take control of their bodies and minds.

Mindfulness increases your confidence because it makes you realise you can do a lot to help yourself when upsetting events and potentially strong, upsetting emotions arise. This 'tool' provides us with the control and security to undertake challenges that we may have shied away from previously.

How does mindfulness differ from relaxation?

The potential difference is one of intent. With relaxation you may be 'switching off' the mind whereas during mindfulness you 'switch on' to yourself and become alert to what is happening. By standing back and observing what is happening in this present moment we may be less wrapped up in our thoughts and feelings, and separate ourselves from them. In mindfulness one can see, as Linehan (1993b) suggests, that a thought is just a thought and an emotion is a set of physical sensations. The recognition that, although not necessarily pleasant, they are not going to harm you can bring about a sense of calmness as you can stand back from considering all the worries of the past, present and future.

Origins of mindfulness

Although mindfulness originated from Buddhist meditation it is not a religious practice. It can be important to mention this to some who may be reluctant to participate as they are not religious, or hold another belief. Instead, it is a method of mental training. You do not have to remain in complete silence, perform it for long periods or sit crossed-legged on the floor. As the Dalai Lama has said, Buddhist monks carry out similar tasks to most of us. The difference is that when they **eat** they just **eat**, when they **walk** they concentrate on **walking**. How many of us eat dinner in front of the television at the same time as talking to a friend? Buddhist monks purposefully direct their attention to the task involved.

Jon Kabat-Zinn introduced the concept of mindfulness into healthcare in 1979. Whilst working largely with patients suffering from chronic pain and cancer in Boston, Massachusetts, he identified that mindful meditation could provide considerable relief from suffering. Since then the use of mindfulness has expanded both within and outside healthcare settings.

How to practise

As we have seen, mindfulness means to be aware of what is actually occurring, internally and externally at this present moment in time. This obviously encompasses a range of items: Things we can experience through our senses; Events; Observing actions of others; Emotions; Physical sensations in our body; Thoughts; Mindful breathing (useful as we always have our breath with us); Everyday mindfulness (e.g. being mindful as we go about our daily tasks).

When practising, it is best to focus upon one rather than all of these and to do so for a couple of minutes, extending the time as you continue to practise. Some clients prefer some types of exercise (for example focusing on a concrete object) whereas some prefer bringing their awareness to their thoughts or breathing. It is useful, therefore, to try a variety of different exercises. Also, whereas some find focusing on a concrete object easier to start with, this changes as they become more experienced. The aim is to be mindful of whatever is effective and useful to you.

Activity 4.2   *Critical thinking*

As you practise the exercises included within this chapter, make notes on these questions.

- Which type of exercise do you find most helpful?
- Does this differ from day to day and when coping with different experiences?
- Has it changed as you become more experienced with using mindfulness?
- Do your preferred mindfulness exercises match those of a colleague/friend?

Teaching clients mindfulness skills often starts by talking them through the exercise to help focus their attention. There are written exercises that clients may find useful and a range of mindfulness CDs and downloads from the internet. As the aim is for clients to practise skills alone at home teachers also, towards the end of courses, provide unstructured mindfulness opportunities to generate a discussion on how to implement mindfulness without a facilitator or teacher there. The aim, at the end of the day, is for them to be able to select and use mindfulness independently within their daily lives and for them to develop confidence in their ability to do this.

Case study

Lisa has practised mindfulness and says, 'I have found knowing I can confidently use this skill in a variety of difficult situations comforting and having the confidence itself (that I can use a skill which proves helpful) has enabled me to cope more effectively with a variety of situations'.

'Having undertaken dialectical behavioural therapy (DBT) I have followed Linehan's (1993b) guide to mindfulness which I feel provides a useful structure to undertaking mindfulness practice. She suggests the "what" and "how" with the first explaining what to do and the latter how to do it (see Table 4.1). There is no right or wrong way to perform mindfulness though'.

What skills	How skills
Observe	Non-judgementally
Describe	One-mindfully
Participate	Effectively

Table 4.1: Linehan's what and how skills

Remember a central concept of mindfulness is to be non-judgemental. Therefore judging whether we are performing the technique 'properly' is just going to give us something else to make judgements on! The aim is for you to develop the most effective technique that allows you personally to be mindful.

Observing

Observing refers to 'standing back' and looking at/experiencing what is happening without labelling it or trying to explain it. Observation is the key word here. You consciously observe an object or your thoughts and feelings rather than getting consumed by them.

For example when observing an object such as a flower, a stone, or a favourite object.

What information can you gain through your senses about the object? Move through them one by one.

Imagine you have come across the object for the first time and attempt to observe it from a new perspective.

Concept summary: Practice 1 – mindfulness of a raisin

I'd like to invite you to take part in a mindfulness exercise involving a raisin. The main aim of this exercise is for us to practise observing the raisin using our senses. Throughout I would like you just to observe and avoid the temptation to put words onto/describe what you are experiencing. This may be an exercise you have undertaken before. If you notice yourself feeling this and perhaps having judgements about performing the exercise I would like you to notice these before we start and try to let them go. I would like us to undertake this exercise as if we are experiencing the sensations involved for the first time.

Holding: Take the raisin and hold it in the palm of your hand. Observe what it feels like as you hold it. Is it light or heavy? Does it feel moist or dry?

Seeing: Take the time to really look at it. Imagine you have never seen one before. Look at it with great care and full attention. Let your eyes explore every part of it from one end to the other. Examine the highlights where the light shines, the folds and ridges.

You may notice the urge to bite into the fruit. If you do so then just notice this urge and observe what it feels like to sit with this urge rather than to follow it.

Touching: Turn the raisin over in your fingers and explore its texture. How does it feel?

Smelling: Now hold it beneath your nose. What does it smell of?

(continued)

(continued)

Placing: Slowly take the raisin towards your mouth and notice how your hand and arm know exactly where to put it. If you feel able bite a piece of raisin. Without chewing simply explore the sensation of having it on your tongue. Gradually begin exploring the object with your tongue,

When you are ready consciously take a bite and notice any tastes that it releases into your mouth. Feel the texture as your teeth bite into it. Continue slowly chewing it. Take another bite if you need to. As you swallow the fruit see if you can follow the sensations of swallowing. Notice how your tongue pushes it towards the back of your mouth and how your mouth prepares to swallow it.

Finally spend a few moments observing any sensations that are in your mouth now it is empty.

When you are ready bring your awareness back into the room around you.

How did you find the exercise?

Did you notice anything different to what you have experienced with a raisin before? (Think how we usually eat raisins in handfuls, or alongside other foods and probably simply swallow them without really paying attention.)

If you had missed these things when 'experiencing a raisin' what other aspects of your life may you be missing out on?

Case study

Lisa found going out into public places challenging and in particular going into shops and waiting in queues. She practised being mindful of a shell given to her by her mother. She started to carry this in her pocket when going out and when becoming agitated practised observing and describing the texture of it. She found this greatly helped her to cope and knowing it was there gave her the confidence to undertake activities she had not previously dared to.

Everyday mindfulness

Fitting mindfulness into a busy everyday life can be a challenge. Incorporating it within your daily activities and being mindful of these provides an excellent reminder and opportunity to practise.

Case study

Sam decided to try mindfully cleaning his teeth as he usually found that when getting ready in the morning he often tried to multitask and his mind was already jumping forward to the day ahead. He found mindfully

cleaning his teeth, through concentrating on one task at once calmed him and his racing mind and enabled him to plan his day more effectively. At night he found it useful in helping 'switch off' and settle to sleep.

Concept summary: Practice 2 – a mindful bath

Try taking a bath mindfully. Observe and then describe the feeling of the water on your skin. Is it hot or cold? Does it feel the same all over your body? Describe the sensations as you wash yourself. Have you any bubbles in the water? What do these smell of? How can you describe them? How can you describe the bar of soap you are using? What sound does the water make as it rushes down the plughole?

For the next week select an activity you perform daily and perform it mindfully each time (e.g. having a bath, cleaning teeth).

- How did you find the exercise? Did you notice anything that you have not done before?
- Did you find your experience and skills in undertaking it mindfully changed over the course of the week?

Observing thoughts and emotions

Another skill in mindfulness is to observe, but not react to, thoughts and feelings (as physical sensations) coming into your mind/body.

Then we 'let them go' – some people find it useful to use guided imagery and imagine them floating away on clouds or see them as signs attached to buses (remembering not to jump on the bus, merely allowing it to pass by!).

Concept summary: Practice 3

Over the next two minutes observe any thoughts, judgements, facts and physical sensations you experience within your body and complete Table 4.2.

Thoughts	Judgements	Facts	Physical sensations

(continued)

(continued)

- How did you find undertaking the mindfulness activity?
- What do you notice about what you wrote in the table above? Does any of it surprise you?
- Do you think any of the above could influence your feelings/emotions?
- How easy did you find it merely to list the above and not respond to any of it?
- Try the exercise again and try to 'let go' of any thoughts/judgements.

Describing

This involves putting words or labels onto what we observe. For example, we may describe what we experience through our senses about an object; when undertaking a task such as washing up we may describe the texture of the bubbles, the smell of the detergent and the sound of the crockery.

Participating

This refers to 'diving in'; being completely absorbed and totally engaging in an activity. It means participating in what you are doing with your mind and body together; not allowing your body to be involved in one activity whilst your mind is elsewhere.

Concept summary: Practice 4

Next time you are eating a meal pretend you are eating for the first time.

Ensure there are no other distractions.

Did you observe anything new?

Marsha Linehan's 'how skills'

Marsh Linehan describes three ways in which we might be mindful: non-judgementally, one-mindfully and effectively. Let's look at these in turn.

Non-judgementally

How often do we evaluate and judge ourselves, others, our feelings and responses? Perhaps we decide whether something is right or wrong? Good or bad? Should or should not have happened? Judgements, in themselves, are perhaps an inevitable part of life and, at times, can be useful. Judging that we were perhaps unkind when talking to someone can help us to say sorry and perhaps repair a friendship. At other times judgements can be unhelpful and trigger overwhelming emotions.

> ### Case study
>
> *A month ago Toby had promised to take his friend James to the cinema the following Friday as a late birthday treat. He had forgotten and asked Simon instead. When they arrived at the cinema he saw James and suddenly remembered the invitation. James was with another group of friends and despite seeing Toby completely ignored him. Toby suddenly remembered the invitation and felt guilty. His mind jumped to the fact he had forgotten James's birthday in the first place and the guilt grew. He felt sad as he had wanted to spend time with James. James's reluctance to acknowledge him expanded the guilt and sadness further and feelings of anger rose … how dare he ignore him …*

As the example above suggests Toby was already feeling guilty. The judgements he made about himself heightened this guilt to an unbearable level and added secondary emotions of anger and sadness.

Mindfulness encourages a non-judgemental approach. As McKay et al. (2007) state, if we are busy judging something our mind is being occupied by this and we are not truly in the present moment (as mindfulness calls for).

Attempting to be completely non-judgemental is hard and when teaching groups we often discuss that noticing we are judging can lead to further judgements about ourselves (we judge ourselves unfavourably for judging!). What may be more realistic is to notice we are judging and 'work on letting this judgement go' before turning our awareness back to the mindfulness activity. After all the actual noticing of our judgements and being able to step back from them demonstrates we are being mindful as we are recognising what thoughts are passing through our mind at this moment in time.

When Lisa, from the case studies, notices herself using phrases such as *shouldn't have, mustn't have* and notices the impact they are having on how she is feeling, Lisa finds it useful to rephrase the situation mindfully by simply describing factually what is going on. How Lisa is feeling about herself often changes significantly after this.

Concept summary: Practice 5 – sketching a horse

How judgemental do you think you are on a scale of 0 to 10? Think of what you say to yourself if you make a mistake.

- Take three minutes and sketch a horse.
- Did any judgements pass through your mind (e.g. I can't draw!, I'm useless!)?
- How did you feel? What emotions, if any, did the exercise result in?
- Did you find your mind jumping to consider other times when you may not necessarily have been pleased with your performance?

One-mindfully

This refers to focusing all your mind and awareness on the current moment – it refers to how we are to participate. When watching my son play football it is obvious that he is not just physically participating in kicking the ball – his mind and body are working as one and he is totally engaged in the activity.

Effectively

This is Linehan's (1993b) last 'how' skill. She refers to this as focusing upon what works and throwing effort into doing what is needed in the actual situation rather than a situation we wish we were in or being more concerned with being right, or feeling good. The phrase 'cutting off your nose to spite your face' has often been applied to this. By practising a mindful, non-judgemental approach this can open our awareness to what is actually happening rather than what we perceive to be happening and assist us in using this skill.

Does your mind wander?

> ### Case study
>
> *During a group where participants were asked to be mindful of sounds in the room around them, Jane reported that her mind had wandered to other things 20 times during a two-minute period. She was disheartened by this and asked what she was doing wrong.*

During these exercises you may find your mind wandering to other things. This does not mean you are not succeeding in being mindful. The fact you noticed your mind has wandered actually demonstrates you are paying complete awareness. One psychologist Lisa worked with described your mind as being like a puppy. It likes to run off and explore! The key to mindfulness is to notice your mind has wandered and to bring it back to the task in hand. Instead of 'failing' Jane was actually demonstrating how mindful she is as she was aware her mind had drifted and was able to bring it back to the task in hand. As for training a puppy this takes practice, practice and more practice!

How long should you practise these exercises for?

There is no right answer to this but as with any exercise it may be most effective to practise for short periods of time (e.g. a minute) to start with and then gradually build up. Rezek (2012) and Williams and Penman (2011) suggest practising for a few minutes each day rather than having a longer session less frequently may be more beneficial. Some people set an alarm or write a note in their diary to remind them to practise. As practising mindfulness when performing everyday tasks can be useful, setting yourself an hour where you are mindful over every task you perform is a good challenge. Lisa now regularly practises this way and has noticed the calmness and clarity of thought it brings her.

It is often easier, as with all skills, to practise them when you are relatively calm rather than trying to practise at times when your anxiety is raised. Lisa additionally finds, through mindfulness, she has become more aware of sensations within her own body, recognises the signs of stress and anxiety earlier and is therefore able to instigate some mindfulness practice at this stage rather than waiting until her emotions have reached a high intensity.

Why knowledge of mindfulness is useful to nurses

Mindfulness is increasingly being used within mental health settings. Although you may not directly be involved in teaching the skill to clients, being able to practise with them, or answer any questions they may have, is important.

Mindfulness is for all! You need to experience mindfulness for yourself. Practice it and see if you notice whether it has any impact on your own life. When teaching groups of clients it is clearly apparent which professionals are really passionate about the skill and who uses it within their life. From personal experience this undoubtedly increases an individual's motivation to learn!

Potential positive effects of mindfulness

Studies have demonstrated that regular practisers are happier and more contented than the average. Mindfulness has proved to improve reaction times and memory (useful in revising for exams!). Mindfulness has been shown to boost the immune system and help fight off colds and 'flu. Regular practisers have been found to enjoy more fulfilling relationships with others.

Uses of mindfulness in mental health settings

Psychological therapies

Mindfulness is a central concept in DBT (Linehan, 1993b) initially developed for BPD; mindfulness-based stress reduction (MBSR); and mindfulness-based cognitive therapy (MBCT).

In major depression: studies (Teasdale et al., 2000) have proven mindfulness is effective at reducing the risks of experiencing a further major depressive episode. The National Institute for Health and Care Excellence (NICE, 2009) has now recommended MBCT for those with a history of three or more episodes of depression. Godfrin and Van Heeringen (2010) found mindfulness reduces the risk of relapse from 68 to 30 per cent for those taking medication as well. Farb et al. (2010) showed that people completing an eight-week MBCT course and stopping medication did as well as, or better than, those remaining on medication.

In drug and alcohol addiction, Zgierska (2010) highlights seven randomised control trials demonstrating improvement. It is proving effective in helping people stop smoking. It also helps people with post-traumatic stress disorder: Quantum (2014) describes how using mindfulness can reduce the trauma of flashbacks by helping them recognise them for what they are and standing back from them.

In eating disorders, mindfulness can help increase sense of control in clients with anorexia nervosa. Kristeller and Hallett (1999) demonstrated it can reduce binge eating.

In psychosis, Abba et al. (2008) undertook a study with 16 participants to identify how mindfulness may help those experiencing psychotic episodes. They advocated mindfulness is effective in helping individuals relate differently to the experiences through helping them ground themselves, allowing voices, thoughts, and images to come and go without reacting or struggle and through reclaiming power by accepting both themselves and the experience. People describe how mindfulness assists them in separating themselves from the auditory or visual hallucinations they are experiencing and in so doing reduces the distress caused by them and assists them in retaining an element of control.

Other uses

Mindfulness can be helpfully used in childbirth. Patients with chronic pain can also use mindfulness with advantage; Grossman et al. (2004) suggest mindfulness may help people separate the physical sensations associated with chronic pain from the often catastrophic thinking that occurs alongside and in so doing increase their coping.

Mindfulness has been shown to help people with cancer recognise that although the disease and associated stress play roles in their lives they can still maintain control and enjoy aspects of their lives.

Mindfulness in children

Mindfulness has proven to be highly effective in cases of attention deficit hyperactivity disorder (ADHD) and in helping children and their families cope with challenging behaviour. It has also been proven in helping children cope with exam stress, get to sleep, manage anger, deal with difficult relationships, improve their performance in sports and handle the increasingly stressful pace and pressure that adolescence sometimes brings. Lisa has experienced the pleasure of going into a sixth form college and facilitating mindfulness classes to teenagers pre-examinations. Feedback from them has been that it helps them concentrate fully on the task in hand and increases their overall sense of control. Goldie Hawn's (2011) book is largely based upon introducing mindfulness to children and family life. Lisa has seen the benefits in her own children and also seen how much they have enjoyed the exercises.

Exploring mindfulness further

On placement it may be possible to participate in a mindfulness group. Lots of teams have started to conduct short mindfulness exercises for staff at the start of the day or at meetings. There are lots of courses you can undertake (e.g. an MBSR course which is an eight-week course, two hours a week). Some universities are offering such courses to students. The Oxford Mindfulness Centre website details both local and national courses. There are additionally online courses you can undertake. The further reading at the end of this chapter also includes both theoretical and more practically orientated materials.

Additional mindfulness exercises to try

Concept summary: Practice 6 – mindful breathing

There are a wide variety of mindfulness exercises involving breathing. It is a highly useful tool as we have it with us all the time and breathing is often altered at times of extreme emotion. Focusing upon it can therefore be useful in assisting us to regulate it and can be very calming.

Mindful breathing:

- Ensure you are in a comfortable position either sitting, standing or lying down.
- Bring your awareness to your breath as it moves in and out of the body. You may find it helpful to concentrate on the sensation of the air moving in and out of your nostrils or, by placing your hand on your abdomen, feeling it rising and falling.
- You may notice mild sensations of stretching as the abdomen gently rises with each in breath and falls with each out breath.
- Try not to alter your breathing in any way. Just pay attention to the air entering and leaving your body.

Concept summary: Practice 7 – mindful body scan

The following exercise, which focuses upon you observing and describing sensations within your body, may be useful in helping a person to ground themselves and is an exercise the author uses on a frequent basis. Some clients find though that a significant proportion of their time is focused upon them looking inwards and that such an exercise exacerbates their distress further by encouraging them to do this on an even greater basis.

- Find a comfortable position for yourself whether sitting or lying down.
- Start with your feet. Observe and describe the sensations of your feet touching your socks and shoes and pressing against the floor. Wriggle your toes and describe the sensations that you can feel.
- Move your attention to your legs. Notice any tension you feel within them.

(continued)

(continued)

- Progress your attention to your buttocks. Observe the pressure of your bottom as it presses against the floor or the chair.
- Move your awareness to your abdomen. Describe any sensations you can feel within it. Place your hand on your abdomen and become aware of your abdomen rising and falling as you breathe in and out.
- Progress to your back. Notice any twisting or bending of your spine and observe and describe any sensations you feel in your back and your shoulders. Are they hunched or relaxed?
- Move your attention to your hands and arms. Observe any tension and notice whether your hands are clenched or relaxed and where they are placed in relation to the rest of your body.
- Draw your awareness to any sensations you are experiencing within your neck. Moving to your head notice any tension in any parts of your face. Observe and describe any tastes you are experiencing within your mouth and any smells you can sense. Observe the feeling of the air moving into and out of your nostrils.
- Finally briefly scan your whole body moving from your head to your toes and notice any changes that you may have experienced as you have undertaken this exercise.

How did you feel undertaking the exercise?

What did you notice within your own body?

Do you feel any different after to before undertaking the exercise?

Concept summary: Practice 8 – mindfulness of blowing bubbles

I would like to invite you to participate in a mindfulness exercise in relation to blowing bubbles.

Before you open them I would like you to feel the container. *How does it feel in your hands? Cool? Smooth?*

Then gently unscrew the cap. *How does it feel to be opening the bubbles? Are you noticing the ridges in the cap? Do you feel excited to be beginning this activity?*

Dip the wand into the bubble mixture and slowly withdraw it. Notice the different colours in the swirls of liquid trapped within the wand. Hold it up to the light and notice how the liquid moves.

Allow a small amount of liquid to drip onto your hand. Describe what it feels like. You may find yourself noticing whether you like or dislike this. If you do, recognise this as a judgement, notice this and then let it go.

Dip the wand into the mixture again and when you are ready start blowing bubbles. Are there many bubbles? Are they large or small? Do the bubbles move a long way from the wand or do they fall to the ground just in front of you. You may find your mind wandering. If you do notice that it has wandered then bring your full attention back to the task of blowing bubbles.

Observe and describe the colours in the bubbles. Are they the same throughout or different? Describe any sounds you hear as the bubbles burst on the floor. Do the bubbles burst straight away or do they sit on the floor for a short time before popping?

You may be aware of others blowing bubbles around you and make judgements about whether your bubbles are smaller or larger than yours or about your or someone else's bubble-blowing ability. If you find yourself doing this just notice it then bring your mind back to the task of blowing bubbles. There is no right or wrong way to blow bubbles or to participate in this activity.

When you are ready I would like you to replace the wand into the bubble pot and screw the lid on.

What did you notice when you were undertaking the exercise?

How to select a mindfulness exercise

The most appropriate focus of a mindfulness activity is whatever you or the client find to be most effective. Often clients find a mindfulness exercise that encourages them to focus upon a concrete object or event the easiest to commence with, becoming more skilled at using more abstract ones (e.g. mindful body scan, being mindful of thoughts) as they gain more practice. Some though find the reverse to be true. It may also depend upon where you are. If you are in the midst of something it may not be appropriate to stop and focus upon an object so turning your complete awareness to the activity you are undertaking or your breath may be most effective. It is useful for clients and yourselves to try a variety of exercises and 'test them out' for themselves.

Chapter summary

Mindfulness is becoming an increasingly used technique both within and outside the healthcare arena. Within mental healthcare it is being used to empower clients to take an active role in assisting the daily challenges they face when dealing with a mental health problem. Although the concept may initially appear easy to grasp it is challenging to learn and requires constant practice with the associated motivation to continue. There are a wide variety of differing mindfulness exercises which have been included within this chapter as differing ones may be appropriate for various situations and individuals may find a particular type most beneficial for them. It is hoped that nurses reading this chapter will practise the technique themselves and recognise the benefit that it may bring to their own lives.

Activities: brief outline answers

As the majority of practice opportunities encourage the student to make their own reflections and draw their own conclusions, those reached within the activities will differ for various individuals. This epitomises the concept of mindfulness. The outline answers have therefore not been provided. The author would encourage nurses to discuss their findings with fellow nurses and healthcare professionals who are familiar with mindfulness to gain another person's insight into the experience.

Further reading

Alidina, S (2010) *Mindfulness for Dummies.* Chichester: John Wiley and Sons.

Heaversedge, J (2010) *The Mindful Manifesto: How doing less and noticing more can help us thrive in a stressed out world.* London: Holly House.

Both books are useful, practical introductory texts.

Useful websites

www.dbtselfhelp.com

www.oxfordmindfulness.org

These websites have been suggested as they include up-to-date information on mindfulness, a range of mindfulness exercises and courses nurses can undertake to develop their skills further.

Chapter 5
Low intensity cognitive behavioural therapy interventions

Simon Grist, Peter Bullard and Janine Ward

NMC Standards for Pre-registration Nursing Education

This chapter will address the following competencies:

Domain 1: Professional values

4.   All nurses must work in partnership with service users, carers, groups, communities and organisations. They must manage risk, and promote health and wellbeing while aiming to empower choices that promote self-care and safety.

4.1. Mental health nurses must work with people in a way that values, respects and explores the meaning of their individual lived experiences of mental health problems, to provide person-centred and recovery-focused practice.

Domain 2: Communication and interpersonal skills

6.   All nurses must take every opportunity to encourage health-promoting behaviour through education, role modelling and effective communication.

6.1. Mental health nurses must foster helpful and enabling relationships with families, carers and other people important to the person experiencing mental health problems. They must use communication skills that enable psychosocial education, problem solving and other interventions to help people cope and to safeguard those who are vulnerable.

Domain 3: Nursing practice and decision-making

4.   All nurses must ascertain and respond to the physical, social and psychological needs of people, groups and communities. They must then plan, deliver and evaluate safe, competent, person-centred care in partnership with them, paying special attention to changing health needs during different life stages, including progressive illness and death, loss and bereavement.

4.1. Mental health nurses must be able to apply their knowledge and skills in a range of evidence-based psychological and psychosocial individual and group interventions to develop and implement care plans and evaluate outcomes, in partnership with service users and others.

Low intensity interventions and how they evolved

Cognitive behavioural therapy (CBT) has grown in strength from the pioneering work of therapists such as Aaron Beck in the 1960s. Cognitive behavioural therapy is now the dominant therapeutic model in the world of evidence-based psychological therapies. The strength of the evidence base has led it to become the primary choice for healthcare settings where evidence base is considered essential to provide the best treatment for patients, for example the National Institute for Health and Care Excellence (NICE) in the UK. While it might be the primary choice it must be remembered that it will not work for all and that patient choice must also be considered when deciding on the therapeutic model used.

Low intensity CBT is a relatively new development in psychotherapy terms, having first been written about and developed at the beginning of this century, relating to the concept of stepped care, and specifically that CBT should be offered both at a less intensive and more intensive level (Bennett-Levy et al., 2010). The Improving Access to Psychological Therapies (IAPT) initiative in England firmly put low intensity CBT on the map.

So what exactly is low intensity CBT? Very broadly the purpose of low intensity CBT is to increase access to evidence-based psychological therapies to improve wellbeing and mental health on a broad community basis using the least restrictive interventions to create the most benefit (Bennett-Levy et al., 2010). When considering this in the context of stepped care this allows low intensity CBT to mainly treat those with mild to moderate psychological disorders, whereas those with more severe disorders are treated with high intensity CBT (how we traditionally think of CBT). Bennett-Levy et al. (2010) suggest that low intensity CBT will demonstrate the following guiding principles:

- reduced contact time with the patient; either by fewer and shorter sessions, or through the use of groups, or facilitation for self-help (i.e. guided self-help);
- using practitioners specifically trained to deliver low intensity CBT, who may not have a formal health profession qualification or who do not hold high intensity CBT qualifications;
- use less intensive CBT resources, e.g. bite-sized pieces, self-paced;
- provide quicker access to psychological therapies, and specifically CBT.

Low intensity CBT is underpinned by basic CBT principles that are delivered through a range of modalities (face to face, telephone, groups and internet) and are generally simple and brief. The principles of guiding the patient with the use of self-help materials, the use of between session work (homework), and extensive use of monitoring to assess and evaluate progress form the basis for CBT. The specific interventions that are used are covered in more detail later in this chapter, including behavioural activation (BA), cognitive restructuring (CR), exposure therapy and problem solving.

Low intensity cognitive behavioural therapy and mental health nursing

While it was not developed to be in secondary care, there is a movement and growing evidence base for the use of low intensity CBT in secondary care settings in the treatment of anxiety and depression. The rationale for potential use in secondary care is focused on functionality, in that many patients with severe and enduring mental health problems commonly have comorbid anxiety and depression. There are a number of advantages in this approach to severe and enduring mental health patients, including that the sessions tend to be shorter, therefore benefiting patients who may struggle with concentration over longer periods of time. The less burdensome nature of the interventions and the self-help element mean that the interventions as a whole are not designed to be complex and can therefore be easily grasped by those who may suffer with varying degrees of cognitive impairment. The session length and frequency means that these interventions may be well suited to clinics or practitioner-led clinics with patients who have achieved stability but still have functional difficulties that may not be considered severe enough for input from a secondary care CBT therapist.

Activity 5.1   *Critical thinking*

While low intensity CBT has a place in secondary care some adaptations may still need to be made. Compile a list of possible adaptations that may help and improve outcomes for this patient group.

Brief outline answers are provided at the end of the chapter.

Primarily these interventions have their evidence base in anxiety and depression, but within secondary care these may be part of the severe mental health presentation and therefore might not be formally diagnosed. This is where your mental health nursing skills are recognising the impact on functioning and the potential for low intensity CBT to reduce this impact and improve quality of life. While this book serves both as a reminder for those trained and an introduction for those not, it does not substitute for good quality training with low intensity CBT (see useful websites).

We will now look at five of the most commonly used low intensity CBT interventions that are used to help patients with anxiety and depression. These are: BA, CR, exposure therapy, problem solving and sleep hygiene.

Behavioural activation

Behavioural activation focuses on changing behavioural aspects of mood to change the person's emotional state and thoughts through activities that impact positively on the individual (Cuijpers et al., 2007a). It is used for depression and is based on rebuilding a person's routine, pleasurable and necessary activities (NICE, N.I.F.H.A.C.E., 2009). This is because when individuals are depressed or low they often cease previous activities because, for example, they lack energy or pleasure in life (American Psychiatric Association, APA, 2000).

Case study

Toby has been feeling down for the last three months following stress at work. He has stopped going out with his friends and is also struggling to attend work. Toby also cannot find the motivation to keep the house clean. He finds himself thinking there is no point in anything, and that he cannot be bothered as nothing works when he tries.

Each of the symptoms of depression keep the other symptoms going; they reinforce missing activities which may initially give the person in the short term a sense of relief but long term have a detrimental effect. For example the person feels worse that they cannot manage what they used to and feels lower in mood which subsequently impacts on them doing activities (Williams, 2009) (see Figure 5.1).

Activity 5.2   *Critical thinking*

Think about a person you have worked with who suffers from depression. What things had they stopped doing? How might this impact on their life?

Brief outline answers are provided at the end of the chapter.

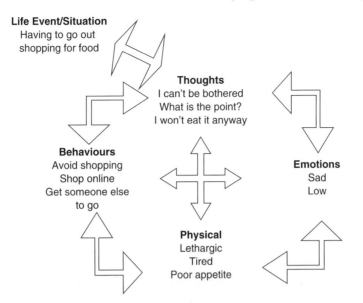

Figure 5.1: Represents the cycle of Toby's low mood. Behavioural activation focuses on behaviour change in the behaviour box

How to implement behavioural activation

Step 1: a baseline diary

Often an individual is given a baseline diary to fill out prior to starting the actual intervention. It records what the person is already doing in their life despite their mood problems. They are often surprised to see how much they are actually achieving. This may boost their mood at the start and encourage motivation (Richards and Whyte, 2011). The baseline diary will also establish a starting point and will show the changes made by BA. This may mean in reaching recovery an individual can see where they have come from and encourage positive reinforcement of building in activities and in themselves (Richards and Whyte, 2011).

Step 2: recording necessary, routine and pleasurable activities

The next step of BA is looking at what activities the individual has stopped doing in their day-to-day life. *Necessary* activities are those which are vital to attend to as otherwise they have significant impact on the person's life, for example paying bills or dealing with difficult situations. *Routine* activities are those which concentrate on day-to-day or week-to-week activities that are part of everyday life, for example cleaning, tidying and washing. *Pleasurable* activities are things the person enjoys doing with others (Richards and Whyte, 2011) (see Table 5.1).

You may wonder why activities are separated into necessary, routine and pleasurable. What benefit or otherwise would this have to the individual? The reason is that the necessary and routine activities are often harder or seem harder than pleasurable ones, but if an individual only does pleasurable things they will not be able to lead a balanced lifestyle. Breaking the activities down allows an individual to be supported in creating a mix of activities. The disadvantage is that highlighting activities that an individual is not doing might make them feel worse in the short term.

Necessary	Stopped going to work
Routine	Cleaning the bathroom Vacuuming the house Weekly shop
Pleasurable	Going to the pub with friends Going to park to walk the dog Playing football on a Tuesday Watching movies with his family

Table 5.1: Shows an example of Toby's necessary, routine and pleasurable activities

Step 3: ordering activities

Now we order the listed activities, from easiest to hardest, while ensuring a mix of necessary, pleasurable and routine activities. This step is important as it ensures that there is a gradual and appreciated approach to reintroducing activities.

Toby ordered his activities like this:

Hardest: Go back to work

  Weekly shopping

Medium: Vacuum the house

  Playing football

  Clean the bathroom

Easy: Go to the park to walk the dog

  Watching films with family

You may notice that not all of Toby's pleasurable activities are easy; you need to look out for a common theme, such as seeing others which people may find hard.

Step 4: planning activities

The next step is to look at planning activities from the list into the week's diary. This should include a mix of pleasurable, necessary and routine activities.

We need to note the 'what, when, where and why' to make the activity specific and objective, as we would in goal setting of any kind. Being specific in setting goals has the effect of encouraging the person to achieve it (Locke et al., 1981). It also has the effect of identifying any barriers or roadblocks that may stop the individual being able to engage in the activity (Westbrook et al., 2011).

Over time the individual should be encouraged to build in all of their activities until they are well and eventually will not need to have the diary as a prompt. Completing the activities should encourage positive reinforcement and improve mood and motivation.

	Monday	Tuesday	Wednesday	Thursday	Friday	Saturday	Sunday
AM: What When Where With whom	Go for a walk in Castle Park with the dog at 10.30 hours on my own		Clean the bathroom at my house at 11.00 on my own				
PM: What When Where With whom							

Figure 5.2: An example BA diary

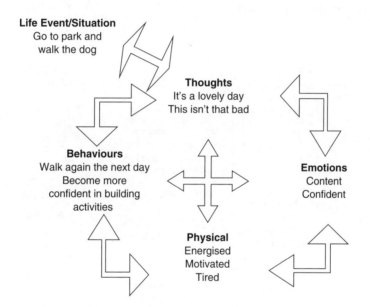

Figure 5.3: Shows how the activities have affected Toby

Over time, Toby may increase his activity levels because of the positive experience of trying activities he had stopped doing. This will take time but may help him to improve his mood and thoughts by changing his behaviours (Hopko et al., 2003).

Summary

Behavioural activation helps an individual to improve their mood by encouraging them to carry out behaviours they have reduced or have avoided. The activities are ordered as pleasurable, routine and necessary and as to their difficulty in starting to do them again. This ensures a balance of activities in the diary and should represent as best as possible their everyday life. Over time thoughts and emotions will change by the positive sense of achievement and reward an individual may get.

Cognitive restructuring

Cognitive restructuring within low intensity CBT is a technique that addresses our negative automatic thoughts (NATs) which occur in situations (Richards and Whyte, 2011).

Negative automatic thoughts occur for all of us in our everyday lives, for example when a friend fails to text you back, or everyone looks at you when you enter a room. You may notice thoughts like 'have I done something wrong?' or 'everyone is looking' or even 'no one likes me'. These thoughts can impact on how you feel, although most people can shake these off and recognise them as just one of those unhelpful thoughts. However, when we are feeling low or anxious our NATs become the fuel of our problem and maintain low mood (Beck, 1963). Figure 5.4 shows how thoughts can maintain our mood.

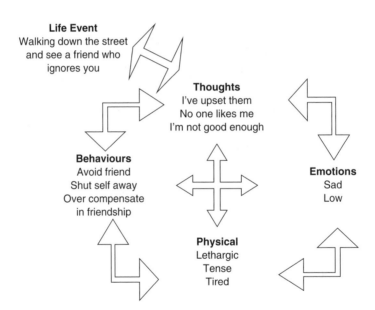

Figure 5.4: The five areas model (Williams and Garland, 2002)

When a person is experiencing NATs, for example 'I'm not good enough', they may start to stay in and avoid things. This may reinforce the thought of 'I'm not good enough' because it limits the person's opportunities to have people around them or enjoy events, and subsequently they may become isolated. This isolation limits opportunities for positive experiences, which feeds and maintains the low mood (Butler and Beck, 1995). If this goes on, over time the person will build up evidence for these NATs, as it is more likely that situations will arise where they respond in an unhelpful way, and therefore the cycle of low mood continues (Williams, 2009).

Recognising negative automatic thoughts in different disorders

Cognitive restructuring in low intensity CBT is typically used with depression, panic disorder and simple phobia (NICE, N.I.F.H.A.C.E., 2009, 2011). However different disorders can be associated with different NATs. Some examples are shown in Table 5.2.

Disorder	Example of NATs
Depression/Low mood	I'm not good enough, everything always goes wrong, what's the point in trying and I can't be bothered.
Gad	'What if …' thoughts about life situations usually out of the person's control. Worries about life and day-to-day things with no specific topic.
Social phobia	Everyone is watching me, I'm being judged, I may make a fool of myself.
OCD	I must do this to stop this [thought, thing or action].
Health anxiety	I might have cancer, I may be ill.
Panic	I'm going to faint, I'm going to have a heart attack, or I'm going to die.
Specific phobia	Thoughts about the object or thing feared.

Table 5.2: NATs in various mental health disorders

Case study

Theresa often finds herself thinking she is no good for anything. She will be at work and anything that colleagues say can make her think she is no good. It happens in her relationship too. Theresa cannot shake the thought and it makes her feel very sad and unconfident.

We will use Theresa's case to illustrate how CR works.

How to implement cognitive restructuring

The principle of CR is to get the person to put their NATs on trial. Because they have gathered evidence to support those thoughts, we need to try to help the individual think about the contrary evidence. First, we help the patient to construct a diary, or chart, like the one shown in Table 5.3.

It is important to note the *situation* which triggers the NAT, as recognising triggers will help in the long term for relapse prevention. The *emotion* is the one that the NAT is causing or impacting upon. This helps the individual understand that the way they think impacts on their mood. Often this helps them understand that they have control over how they feel and how to change their emotional state. Emotions describe how someone feels and are usually one word. Figure 5.5 is an emotion wheel which has a selection of emotional states that may be used.

Situation	Emotion (Intensity 0–100%)	Thought (Belief 0–100%)	Evidence for	Evidence against	Revised thought (0–100%)	Emotion (Intensity 0–100%)
Work meeting and someone interrupts	Low confidence 60% Low 20%	I'm not good enough 70% No one cares what I think 50% I never have anything important to say 40%	I have been interrupted, no one cares what I think. Last time someone ignored what I was saying.			

Table 5.3: Theresa's diary

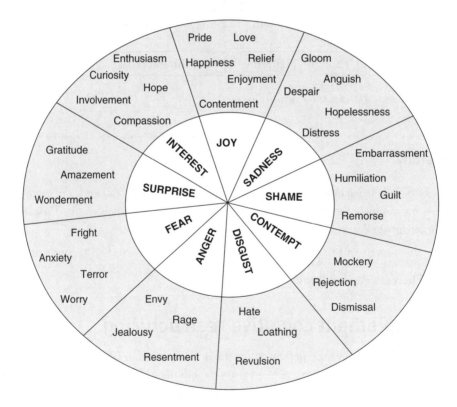

Figure 5.5: An emotion wheel (from www.getselfhelp.co.uk)

Rating the *distress* helps individuals to realise which emotions are closely linked to their problem. It shows the intensity of their feelings and which emotion is strongly linked to their thought. The *thought* column indicates the main thoughts going through an individual's mind; rating the *belief in the thought* helps to identify the thought which is most clearly linked to the emotional state. This is known as the 'Hot Thought' and is the thought which should be restructured.

Activity 5.3   *Critical thinking*

Think about how Theresa may have started to support her NATs. This will form the evidence for a NAT and will underpin why she cannot just let the NAT go as just another thought.

Brief outline answers are provided at the end of the chapter.

The next part of CR looks at finding evidence for and against the thought. It is important to gather the evidence for the thought as the person needs to know what it is that keeps the thought going. To help the evidence against the thought the following questions may be useful.

- What would a friend say?
- If you looked back six months from now, would you think the same way?
- Are you basing what you think on what you feel?
- If you believe it only a certain percentage, what makes up the rest of your belief?

The next step is coming up with a revised thought which should be balanced and counteract the original NAT. This will be rated on how much the person believes in the thought. Creating an alternative balanced thought should impact on the emotion that occurred when thinking the NAT. It may even generate a different emotional state.

Table 5.4 is an example of Theresa's thought diary with the evidence for and against included.

Situation	Emotion (Intensity 0–100%)	Thought (Belief 0–100%)	Evidence for	Evidence against	Revised thought (0–100%)	Emotion (Intensity 0–100%)
Work meeting and someone interrupts	Low confidence 60% Low 20%	I'm not good enough 70% No one cares what I think 50% I never have anything important to say 40%	I have been interrupted, no one cares what I think. Last time someone ignored what I was saying.	I have shared ideas and they have been implemented before. I have led meetings so I must know what I am talking about.	I can deliver my point when he is finished 50% I am ok 60%	Confident 40% Low 10% Relieved 20%

Table 5.4: Theresa's thought diary

Theresa's emotional state has been impacted by the difference in her thoughts and her belief in these thoughts. This may change her behaviours and physical symptoms.

As you may see from the diary, having some doubt in the thought can impact on the emotion. Therefore being able to find evidence against the thought is integral to the intervention. Over time the client's rating of their less negative emotional intensity should increase, and the outcome may help the client to discount their NATs when they pop up (Beck, 1963). Figure 5.6 is an example of how this may be demonstrated in a five areas diagram.

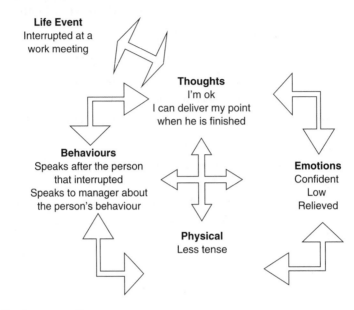

Figure 5.6: The five areas diagram

Summary

Overall CR helps the individual to both disregard and challenge their NATs in situations which should ultimately have an impact on their emotional state. Using CR over time should encourage this to be an automatic process and may help the individual become a balanced thinker and not to accept NATs as truth.

Exposure therapy

Patients with high levels of anxiety often adopt the strategy of avoidance and escape as ways of coping. While this strategy achieves a short-term sense of relief from not having to confront the perceived situation of danger, the longer term impact is much more significant. In adopting these behaviours, patients are teaching themselves that they cannot cope in situations, reinforcing the idea that anxiety is harmful and further reinforcing their lack of confidence. Exposure therapy is a low intensity CBT treatment that helps individuals to tackle their avoidance in a step-by-step approach (Papworth et al., 2013).

Graded exposure or *in vivo* exposure

Before we introduce the steps of this intervention, it is first worth considering the different types of exposure therapy. The low intensity CBT approach is known as 'graded exposure'. This approach lends itself more to the guided self-help nature of low intensity interventions, as collaboration is undertaken between the nurse and patient, then implemented outside of the contact time (low intensity book).

In vivo ('in the living body') exposure fits into the traditional CBT treatment model. With this approach the therapist would be present when the exposure session is undertaken (Westbrook et al., 2011). An example of this would be an individual who has a fear of spiders. The therapist would sit with the patient with a spider present and begin by touching it themselves. They would then support the patient to gradually get closer to the spider and habituate to the anxiety felt in that situation. This requires longer appointments, so is not practised in low intensity settings.

The rationale and psycho-education

Exposure therapy should be introduced with a clear rationale and discussed collaboratively to ensure the patient understands the links between their thoughts, physical symptoms and behaviour. At this point psycho-education around the role of the fight/flight response is also needed to help the patient understand the rationale for exposure therapy.

The fight/flight response

The fight/flight response is in all animal life and can be seen as an internal safety mechanism. Earliest humans, like animals, would have to fight or run in order to survive. In modern society, although we do not live in such primitive circumstances, we still maintain this instinctive response to threat. When an individual is faced with a perceived situation of danger (identified in assessment as the trigger for anxiety) the body releases adrenaline which prepares the body to either fight the situation, or run from it. At this point the body is trying to shuttle oxygenated blood to the main muscle groups in the body and this produces the physical symptoms that patients often live in fear of.

It is important to emphasise that this is a normal response that cannot harm us. The problem is that as we avoid and escape situations, we never learn the response is harmless and the body never gets a chance to feels the anxiety reduce (through the parasympathetic nervous system). Adrenaline can only stay in the body for up to an hour, so these symptoms would naturally reduce if we stayed in the situation long enough.

The idea of the intervention is to gradually expose ourselves to feared situations and remain in them long enough to feel this reduction in anxiety. This process is called habituation and is achieved when an individual no longer feels the anxiety as strongly when confronted with the feared stimulus and it dissipates quicker than it did before (Papworth et al., 2013).

The four rules of graded exposure therapy

1. *Graded*: The analogy of learning to drive can be considered with the first rule. When we learn to drive we do not start on the busiest, fastest, trickiest motorway. This would be overwhelming and likely scare us into not using the car for a good while after. Instead most people start in a car park at a quiet time of day. Once the person feels confident in this situation they may move onto a smaller, quiet road, then progress to somewhere busier.

The same idea can be used for grading exercises. A hierarchy should be developed taking into consideration the final goal, starting point and what exposure tasks will gradually introduce more challenging situations.

2. *Repeated*: As this is an intervention, tasks need to be undertaken and planned in at least four times a week. The more opportunities a patient has to confront anxiety, the more the body has the chance to habituate to the situation.

3. *Timed*: As part of the exercise the patient will rate their SUDS (subjective units of distress 0–100 per cent anxiety) before, during and after the exposure activity has taken place. The patient needs to experience at least a 50 per cent reduction in anxiety from their initial rating for the body to habituate to symptoms. Keep in mind adrenaline dissipates after about one hour, so it is likely 10 minutes in a feared situation will not be enough.

4. *Without distraction*: For the patient to get used to the symptoms of anxiety they need to fully experience the feeling reduce. This can be interrupted if the patient uses distraction techniques. Examples may be quickly going to a nearby toilet for respite from the symptoms, checking or speaking to someone on their phone, or having someone to accompany them to situations. Try and avoid distraction techniques when using exposure therapy and reiterate the rationale if a patient struggles with this.

Activity 5.4   *Critical thinking*

Develop an exposure hierarchy based on the previously discussed principles that would help Sally tackle her anxiety.

Sally, 45, presents with panic and agoraphobia and has for some time avoided being in public places. Sally fears she will have a panic attack and pass out, causing an embarrassing scene. This is having a negative impact on her life as she cannot go out to shop for food or clothing, or to meet up with friends. Sally's worst fear would be going to a busy supermarket on a Saturday.

- What considerations do you need to make when developing the hierarchy?
- What potential barriers may you face when developing the hierarchy?

Exposure task ....

Difficult ....

Medium ....

Easiest ....

....

Brief outline answers are provided at the end of the chapter.

Setting exposure tasks

Exposure tasks based on the hierarchy can be agreed in treatment sessions, or if less time is available, set as a homework task. An important part of the exercise is getting patients to consider their SUDS. The individual rates their anxiety levels before, at the beginning of and after exposure tasks on a scale of 0–100 per cent (100 per cent being as bad as the anxiety can be) (see Figure 5.7). This is an important part of the process as it provides a visual representation of change and helps the patient reflect on their experience more objectively than simply paying attention to how bad the anxiety was initially. Table 5.5 is an exposure planning sheet for a patient with a fear of busy places.

0%	25%	50%	75%	100%
No anxiety		Moderate anxiety		High anxiety

Figure 5.7: Anxiety scale

Date and duration	Exposure task	Anxiety before	Anxiety at beginning	Anxiety after	Comments
Monday 12th at 11 am for 45 minutes	Go to local small corner shop	85 per cent	90 per cent	50 per cent	Really worried at start but forced myself to do it. Felt less anxious after.
Wednesday 14th at 11 am for 40 minutes	Go to local small corner shop	70 per cent	75 per cent	40 per cent	Did not feel anxious for as long a period of time

Table 5.5: An exposure planning sheet

The four exposure principles need to be considered when creating a plan. They must be graded and therefore selected from the appropriate section of the hierarchy, depending where the patient is in treatment. The patient should be asked to plan in at least four tasks in a week to achieve the repetition principle. The tasks must last at least until the anxiety has reduced by half. Avoiding distraction should also be discussed when considering tasks as this may form a barrier to achieving habituation.

Barriers to success in exposure therapy

Barriers in exposure therapy can prevent the patient from getting the most out of treatment. Below are some common barriers that present in treatment which prevent patients from progressing with exposure therapy.

Breaking the graded principle

It is common that patients may think the first task is too simplistic, or are keen to progress through treatment quickly out of frustration with their symptoms. Sometimes patients will jump too far up the hierarchy and report feeling overwhelmed by the scenario. Here it is important to reiterate the rationale and encourage the individual to select an easier exposure task, before habituation is achieved and moving up the hierarchy.

Not enough repetition

Patients may report back in sessions they have completed a task once but on no other occasions. While they should be supported in taking this step, this may also signal avoidance from facing scenarios. At this point discuss the patient's understanding of the rationale and highlight the importance of repetition to help achieve habituation.

Leaving early

If the patient has misunderstood the rationale or is simply overwhelmed by the situation they have faced, when discussing the exposure diary it may be revealed that the individual only stayed in the scenario for 10–15 minutes. Reiterating the time principle is important here and potentially a review of the step in hierarchy.

Avoidance

Avoidance can present in many ways during exposure therapy. Patients may be using distraction techniques such as looking at their phone, going to places with a trusted friend or taking regular trips to the toilet as way of distracting themselves from the anxiety. Here it is important to discuss the patient's understanding of safety behaviours and how these can prevent habituation.

This is not an exhaustive list of problems which may present in exposure therapy; however all are common problems and should be addressed in sessions with the nurse.

Review sessions should include the patient's understanding and progress with the intervention, problem-solving barriers to treatment and setting exposure therapy task goals to complete for the next appointment. The patient's understanding of tasks to take away from the session should be sought at the end of the appointment.

Scenario

You are nursing Rebecca, 24, who has a deep phobia of spiders. Table 5.6 is a completed exposure chart for Rebecca. Rebecca has completed an assessment and first treatment session in which she took away homework to complete four exposure tasks. Rebecca returns the following week presenting as highly anxious and questioning the treatment plan. You need to review the exposure diary and decide what rules of exposure have been broken in observation of the diary. You also need to think about how to work with Rebecca to help her overcome these barriers.

Date and duration	Exposure task	Anxiety before	Anxiety at beginning	Anxiety after	Comments
Monday for 30 minutes	Look at picture of small house spider	80 per cent	85 per cent	75 per cent	
Tuesday for 30 minutes	Look at picture of small house spider	75 per cent	80 per cent	70 per cent	Little less scared this time
Wednesday for 10 minutes	Look at video of spider on internet	80 per cent	85 per cent	85 per cent	Felt too scared watching it and stopped!!!
Friday	Look at video of spider on internet	85 per cent	–	–	Couldn't face it again

Table 5.6: Rebecca's exposure chart

Problem-solving therapy

So often when patients present with mental distress their symptoms are accompanied by problems in their day-to-day life. Some problems may develop because of an inability (or perceived inability) to deal with situations, while others may be the trigger for distress. Problem-solving therapy is evidence based in the treatment of depression (Cuijpers et al., 2007b; Mynors-Wallis et al., 2000) and can also be used for the treatment of anxiety.

Bell and D'Zurilla (2009) suggest individuals with a positive problem-solving orientation are less likely to experience problems with their mental wellbeing than those with a negative problem-solving orientation. Problem-solving orientation is the patient's attitude and behaviour towards problems. Table 5.7 highlights some common features of problem-solving orientation that you may notice when working with individuals.

	Positive problem-solving orientation	Negative problem-solving orientation
Thoughts	'Problems are a challenge but can be solved' 'Problems take time and persistence to overcome' 'If I break problems into small steps they will become easier to manage'	'Problems are overwhelming' 'I can't cope, it's all too much, I can never deal with situations' 'The task is too great'
Behaviour	Makes time to deal with problem and identifies steps required Faces situations Reflects on steps to solving problems and learns for next time	Avoids situations Procrastination Ruminates over problems No planning of ways to resolve issues

Table 5.7: Problem-solving orientation

As we can see, the mindset of the individual with a positive problem-solving orientation leads to behaviours that help to deal with situations and in turn reinforces their positive problem-solving skills. The patient who perceives problems as an unachievable task avoids situations, does not resolve the issue and reinforces their sense of being unable to cope. This in turn reinforces their sense of distress, and maintains worries and symptoms of depression.

> ### Case study
>
> *Eva is a 36-year-old female presenting with depression. She lives on her own with three children. She has experienced recurrent depression for a number of years but recently this has been exacerbated by a number of situational problems. She is finding managing her finances difficult and this is leading to increasing levels of debt. As a consequence she has put on weight through over-eating (which is affecting her self-esteem), is avoiding friends and family and reports struggling with the children. When asked what she has tried so far to tackle the problem, Eva says 'I feel so overwhelmed by everything that I have turned a blind eye and just tried to take each day as it comes'.*

As we can see, Eva is displaying a negative problem-solving orientation. She perceives problems as overwhelming and avoids taking steps to resolving them.

The problem-solving intervention can be broken down into steps and delivered in a way that fits with the contact time between patient and nurse (Bennet Levy et al., 2010). You need to think about the patient's level of motivation, because they will need to commit to doing some brief homework tasks.

Creating insight into problems

Often patients have avoided dealing with problems for so long that they have little insight into what is causing them to feel as they do. A helpful way of gaining perspective and insight is by creating a problem list. This may take up most of the first session spent on problem solving. The list can then be reviewed and items prioritised for the next steps of the intervention. Using Eva as an example, the problem list below begins to break down the contributing factors to her depression.

Eva's problem list:

- debt increasing on credit cards;
- gaining weight;
- feeling unable to see friends and family due to shame around my situation;
- not knowing how much money I have coming in and going out;
- not being able to do things with the children because of finances.

The steps of problem solving

In many cases the contact between nurse and patient will not last long enough to resolve all of the patient's problems (some problems may take many months to resolve). With this in mind it is important the patient learns to use the steps of problem solving so eventually they can apply them without the aid of a professional. There are seven steps to consider, each illustrated using examples from Eva's case.

Step 1: establishing the problem

Together, you need to agree on a problem to focus on. Issues obviously causing the most distress may be prioritised over problems that can be addressed over a longer period of time. Help guide the patient to make a choice using open questioning skills:

'If you could change one thing about your current circumstances, what would that be?'

'Looking at the list, which feels like the greatest priority for you?'

The chosen problem should be made specific. In Eva's case 'money problems' can be made more specific by writing 'increasing credit card debt'. This is a more manageable problem then the initial broader term.

Step 2: listing solutions

As we have seen, the goal of problem solving is not only to resolve issues but also to increase the patient's sense of being able to manage difficulties when they arise. Ask the patient to list as many solutions as they can think of, no matter how strange or unlikely they are to resolve the problem. This should be patient-led but supported with your ideas.

Eva's solutions:

- ask to borrow money from parents;
- speak to credit card company about the problem;
- speak to debt advice company about manageable repayments;
- win the lottery;
- get a part-time job.

Step 3: reviewing solutions

The patient should now review each solution for its pros and cons. Using a table like Eva's (Table 5.8) is an easy way of doing this. There may be a number of pros and cons for each example but engaging in this process helps better inform the patient's decision over how they will try and resolve problems.

Pros	Cons
Help manage repayments	They may limit my spending
Help plan my income and outgoings	May be able to do even less with children
Help me understand my situation	
May feel more in control of situation	

Table 5.8: Solution: Speak to debt advice company

The review process can take some time if there are many solutions. This could be set as a piece of homework to complete between contacts.

Step 4: choosing a solution

Once all solutions have been considered you should collaborate with the patient over their chosen approach. This should be guided and the pros and cons of each solution considered. If there is obvious risk to the patient or others with one of the solutions you should discuss your concerns.

Step 5: action plan

Now you can look at the actions needed to implement the solution, with the following questions:

When will the patient make time to implement the solution?
Who will the patient need to contact/have present to action the solution?
Where will the solution take place?

It is important to have a clear picture of what the patient is going to do. The nurse can establish this using open questions:

'Just so I can make sure I have a clear understanding, what are you going to do after today's contact?', *'Can you explain your understanding of the plan?'*

Some patients may benefit from using an activity diary to schedule in time to implement the plan.

Step 6: putting solution into action

This is the patient's responsibility to complete between contacts. They carry out the plan agreed to tackle the agreed problem.

Step 7: review

Once the action plan has been carried out, the nurse and patient review the outcome. It should be noted that some problems may take several solutions to resolve. For example, in Eva's case resolving her debt problems may require several actions:

- speak to debt management company;
- speak to credit card company;
- meet with her bank to create a balance sheet of incomings and outgoings;
- discuss childcare with her family to free her to look for a part-time job.

The nurse should reflect on the process with the patient. If the solution did not work, review why and then return to the solutions list, choosing another to attempt.

Once the problem has been resolved, the patient can return to the problem list and begin to tackle other issues. You need to repeat the approach to develop and reinforce problem-solving skills.

Sleep hygiene

Sleep problems can contribute to development of mental health problems as much as they can maintain them. While the pathology of disorders can differ significantly across the broad spectrum of mental health problems faced by a nurse, this one symptom is commonly present and observed. In the NICE guidelines for depression (2012), sleep hygiene is recommended as an intervention which should be offered to all patients. It should not be discounted either in the case of anxiety, where so often patients are kept up until the early hours worrying about life situations and physical symptoms.

Sleep hygiene is a method used to promote more restful sleep, feeling refreshed on waking and having more energy in the day time. Like the previous low intensity interventions it is delivered in steps, with the nurse supporting the individual to implement changes.

Identifying the sleep problem

Take time to assess the type of sleep problem experienced by the patient. This might include the following problems.

Problems falling asleep

The patient may report lying in bed for hours unable to get off. They may be tossing and turning, thinking about the day's events and what may happen tomorrow. Clock watching may have become a habit.

Problems staying asleep

Staying asleep may have become a problem for the patient, waking up after only a few hours, falling in and out of sleep, or simply waking earlier than they would like.

Problems with sleeping too much

Some patients may report the quality of their sleep is so bad, they spend more time in the day making up for it. This is not helpful as the sleep they are getting is likely of poor quality, leaving them tired after naps or short periods of rest.

Feeling tired in the day

It is common that patient report sleeping enough but still feel tired in the day time. This may be an indication that the quality of sleep they are getting is not good. Assessing influences on poor sleep quality is important here. Factors may include life stresses, problems in the environment or substance use.

Medical problems

Along with a psychological assessment of sleep the patient should also be asked about any medical conditions that may influence sleep. It may then be helpful to support them in consulting the correct health professional.

Behaviour	Monday	Tuesday	Wednesday	Thursday	Friday	Saturday	Sunday
Activity during day	Little activity – walked to local shop						
Activity before bed	Watched TV						
Caffeine	5 cups of tea						
Alcohol	2 glasses of wine an hour before bed						
Time spent in bed	10pm–7am						
Time spent awake in bed	Took 4 hours to get to sleep						
Hours slept	5						
Energy levels (0 being exhausted and 10 fully refreshed)	3						

Table 5.9: Example of sleep diary (with one day completed)

Getting a clear picture

One of the most helpful ways of establishing a patient's sleep pattern and behaviours is to ask them to complete a sleep diary. There are many examples of sleep diaries and the one in Table 5.9 is not exhaustive of information that may be helpful to ascertain. A sleep diary can be used to identify areas where patients can set goals for change.

Sleep hygiene advice

Discuss sleep hygiene and give advice when you have contact with the patient, and offer further literature. The patient may benefit from selecting one or two areas to change at first, and building on this over the course of contact.

Research summary

Westbrook et al., in their *An Introduction to Cognitive Behaviour Therapy: Skills and Applications* (2011) describe several areas of advice on sleep.

Education: It is not uncommon to hold beliefs about sleep which can exacerbate the problem. A discussion around the patient's perception of 'how much is enough sleep?'

can reveal the person's expectations do not fit with the reality of what they need. The average amount of sleep required for working age adults is between 7 and 9 hours (activity depending). As we pass the age of 65 the need reduces to 5–7 hours.

Have a set time to sleep: The body runs on a 24-hour natural clock (also known as the circadian rhythm). This can become disrupted when feeling unwell and lead to a variety of times when the patient attempts to sleep. It is more helpful in the case of sleep problems to have a set time to sleep and wake up. This can help to establish a routine and a consistent time when the patient begins to feel tired. Having a routine can help to establish a sleep time, for example planning to a have bath or using the last half an hour before bed to listen to relaxing music.

Picture and sound: In modern Western society many households have TVs, computers, laptops or smartphones ready to play music and films/programmes at the touch of a button. This is not helpful in the environment where the individual wishes to sleep as it can promote emotions that prevent us from feeling tired. Removing such stimuli from the sleep environment can promote a sense of restfulness.

Environment: Consider the environment the patient is sleeping in. Temperature is important along with the amount of light in the room. The body produces melatonin, a chemical which helps us to feel tired, when in presence of darkness. Consider if there are bright street lamps or lights on in the house? Does the sun light up the room in the early hours leading to premature waking? If so, problem-solve how to overcome this issue. The comfort of the patient's mattress and pillows can also be a simple but effective consideration.

Taking naps: It is common patients will try and nap during the day to make up for a lack of sleep. While in the short term this may provide some sense of rest, in the longer term it is detracting from the period when they need to achieve quality rest. Initially patients may be reluctant to give up naps. Supporting the individual to reduce the frequency and length of naps can be a good starting point, encouraging no more than 30 minutes at a time. The rationale here is although they will feel more tired in the day without their nap, they are more likely to achieve quality sleep at night.

Alcohol: So often used as an easy way to get off to sleep, while providing a short-term sedating effect, alcohol prevents the brain from entering the deeper stages of sleep which are required to feel refreshed on waking. They may also find themselves taking regular trips to the toilet at night! Patients should be advised to reduce consumption in general and especially before they go to bed. Educating them on the short- and long-term effects can be helpful here.

Turn the clock around: Clock watching can become a maintaining behaviour in the cycle of sleep problems. Often patients worry about the consequence of not getting enough sleep (e.g. 'If I don't sleep for 9 hours I will be terrible at work and unable to function, then I will lose my job and my mortage!!!'), so as the minutes tick by and they become more anxious, they focus more on the clock. This is not helpful as it maintains the negative thought that they cannot sleep. Ask the patient to consider moving the clock so it is not so easy to check.

(continued)

(continued)

Physical activity and lifestyle: Patients often reduce levels of activity when experiencing mental health problems. Physical activity can help increase levels of fatigue so when they come to sleep, they natural fall into a deeper state. Behavioural activation can be used to help gradually build activity levels.

Diet should also be considered. Patients should avoid going to bed excessively full but also starving hungry. Having a snack in the lead up to sleep can help promote tiredness.

Take a break from 'trying' to sleep: When sleep becomes a problem frustration can set in and it is not uncommon that patients will be lying in bed for hours trying to 'force' themselves to sleep. The longer time is spent tossing, turning and allowing frustrating thoughts to build, the less restful the body becomes. One way of breaking this vicious circle is to ask the patient to leave the environment. The bed itself can become associated with anxiety, so a helpful behaviour change can be to leave the bed after 20–30 minutes if sleep has not been achieved. They should consider going somewhere else in the home where they can sit quietly in darkness, until starting to feel tired again.

This scenario may also reveal anxious thoughts about sleep, for example 'If I can't sleep I won't be able to do my job and then I will get fired!' Or 'I won't be able to cope with the children if I do not get my 8 hours'. At this point it may be useful to spend some time engaging cognitive techniques to challenge feared scenarios.

Bringing it all together

Improving the quality of patients' sleep is a collaborative effort. A rationale for change should first be given followed by goal setting. It is important to reiterate changes must be sustained to have an impact and it is unrealistic to expect sleep quality to change in just a few days.

Chapter summary

We have looked at a number of interventions based on CBT theories that can be used with our patients who have anxiety and depression. There is a strong evidence base for the use of these techniques in primary care, and the evidence base in secondary care is beginning to grow, although this is obviously complicated by the more severe mental health problems that tend to be comorbid with anxiety and depression. We have looked at interventions aimed at challenging cognitive biases, CR, and ones aimed at behavioural strategies, BA and exposure therapy. We have also looked at two practically based interventions which can be useful for anybody, but are also a common feature in secondary mental health care patients, namely sleep hygiene and problem solving. While we have given an overview of these interventions as a guide to help they do not aim to replace good quality CBT training and use of these techniques should be supported with high quality CBT specific supervision.

Activities: brief outline answers

Activity 5.1 Critical thinking

Some possible adaptations include:

- more sessions to allow for poor concentration or cognitive impairment;
- breaking sessions and tasks down into smaller sections;
- utilising visual and other learning aids to increase understanding;
- provision of reminder calls for appointments and in-between session tasks;
- enlisting the support of carers and care staff to support patients, especially in earlier stages;
- joint work with primary care team to ensure shared goals and objectives.

Activity 5.2 Critical thinking

There are often common things that individuals with depression do, for example stop going out socially, reduce the housework that they are doing, reduce going anywhere outside their home.

Activity 5.3 Critical thinking

NATs are often supported by life events or occurrences that support the thought. For example if Theresa had been interrupted at work or had had times whereby she thought someone was being negative she may have used this for evidence to support her thoughts.

Activity 5.4 Critical thinking

An easier activity on the hierarchy could be going to her local shop for a newspaper, with a medium difficulty task of going to the supermarket in a quiet time for a couple of items. A difficult one would be doing a full shop at a quiet time with the most difficult being a shop on a busy Saturday morning.

As a practitioner it would be important to consider the impact this is having on Sally, and therefore be empathic. It would also be important to ensure that Sally met the conditions necessary for exposure to be effective (graded, prolonged, timed and without distraction).

Some barriers might be Sally's resistance to the task, not meeting the conditions necessary for the exercise and skipping too far up the hierarchy. It is also important to explore any potential barriers that Sally might identify and therefore remain collaborative.

Further reading

Bennett-Levy, J, Richards, DA and Farrand, P (2010) Low intensity CBT interventions: a revolution in mental health care, in Bennett-Levy et al. (eds) *Oxford Guide to Low Intensity CBT Interventions.* Oxford: Oxford University Press.

This is one of the first low intensity specific texts to be published and as such contains some very useful history and information.

Papworth, M, Marrinan, T, Martin, B, Keegan, D and Chaddock, A (2013) *Low Intensity Cognitive Behaviour Therapy: A Practitioners Guide.* London: Sage.

A later specific low intensity text which is specifically designed for use by a practioner.

Richards, D and Whyte, M (2011) *Reach Out: National Programme Student Materials to Support the Delivery of Training for Psychological Wellbeing Practitioners Delivering Low Intensity Interventions.* London: Rethink.

The standard text for the training of low intensity CBT practitioners.

Westbrook, D, Kennerly, H and Kirk, J (2011) *An Introduction to Cognitive Behaviour Therapy: Skills and Applications,* 2nd edition. London: Sage.

A slightly more advanced CBT text, but still useful in gaining an understanding of the basics.

Useful websites

www.bps.org.uk/careers-education-training/accredited-courses-training-programmes/psychological-wellbeing-practition

This is a source of providers for IAPT low intensity CBT training.

www.getselfhelp.co.uk

A therapist's resource site with a number of useful CBT tools.

www.iapt.nhs.uk

The national website for IAPT, and contains some useful information about IAPT and low intensity CBT.

www.ntw.nhs.uk/pic/selfhelp

A useful website which contains a number of self-help guides

www.phqscreeners.com/overview.aspx?Screener=03_GAD-7

Use this website to download a PDF copy of the GAD-7.

www.phqscreeners.com/overview.aspx?Screener=02_PHQ-9

Use this website to download a PDF copy of the PHQ-9.

www.psychology.tools/download-therapy-worksheets.html

Another useful resource site for therapists

Chapter 6
Why should I get fit? Physical activity as an intervention

Simon Grist

NMC Standards for Pre-registration Nursing Education

This chapter will address the following competencies:

Domain 1: Professional values

5. All nurses must fully understand the nurse's various roles, responsibilities and functions, and adapt their practice to meet the changing needs of people, groups, communities and populations.

Domain 3: Nursing practice and decision-making

Field standard for competence:

Mental health nurses must draw on a range of evidence-based psychological, psychosocial and other complex therapeutic skills and interventions to provide person-centred support and care across all ages, in a way that supports self-determination and aids recovery. They must also promote improvements in physical and mental health and well-being and provide direct care to meet both the essential and complex physical and mental health needs of people with mental health problems.

8. All nurses must provide educational support, facilitation skills and therapeutic nursing interventions to optimise health and well-being. They must promote self-care and management whenever possible, helping people to make choices about their healthcare needs, involving families and carers where appropriate, to maximise their ability to care for themselves.

8.1 Mental health nurses must practise in a way that promotes the self-determination and expertise of people with mental health problems, using a range of approaches and tools that aid wellness and recovery and enable self-care and self-management.

This chapter will address the following ESCs:

Essential skills cluster: Organisational aspects of care

9.   People can trust the newly registered graduate nurse to treat them as partners and work with them to make a holistic and systematic assessment of their needs; to develop a personalised plan that is based on mutual understanding and respect for their individual situation promoting health and well-being, minimising risk of harm and promoting their safety at all times.

18.   Discusses sensitive issues in relation to public health and provides appropriate advice and guidance to individuals, communities and populations for example, contraception, substance misuse, smoking, obesity.

22.   Works within a public health framework to assess needs and plan care for individuals, communities and populations.

Chapter aims

After reading this chapter you will be able to:

- critically evaluate the policy surrounding physical activity;
- demonstrate knowledge of the evidence base around the benefits of physical activity;
- understand the levels of activity that are necessary to benefit both mental and physical health;
- use strategies to help your patients become more active;
- be aware of some of the cautions to physical activity.

Introduction

Physical activity has been a feature of human life since the earliest stages of humankind. It has existed in many different guises and has been called many different things, but essentially it is part of who we are and as such integral to human lives. Back in the early days of humankind it formed a definitive purpose, that of gathering food and the ability to move between areas, be it foraging for plants or hunting animals for meat, and as our societies and knowledge grew, the cultivation of plants or transport from one area to another. However over time as we advanced and became more efficient at extracting resources from the environment our activity levels have fallen (Katzmarzyk, 2010). It is therefore not surprising that we are seeing a rise in obesity, diabetes, cardiovascular disease and other chronic diseases in our societies, despite advances in medical science and technology.

Activity 6.1   *Evidence-based practice and research*

Although there is no policy-level physical activity promotion from the UK government, there is some guidance. For example, there is *Start Active, Stay Active: A Report on Physical Activity from the Four Home Countries' Chief Medical Officers* (Department of Health, DH, 2011b) and the Change4Life campaign (**http://change4life.icnetwork.co.uk**).

Start with these to see what campaigns and guidance are current and local to your geographical area.

As this is based on your own research, no answer is provided.

In this chapter we will be considering why this should be important to us as mental health nurses. We will be looking at the benefits physical activity confers to all of us, regardless of mental or physical health difficulties and how much activity is necessary to provide protection against chronic diseases. We will cover some of the cognitive interventions to support our patients to be more active, including thinking about the barriers that may be raised by them, or us!

The importance of fitness in mental health nursing

As mental health nurses we have a duty of care and responsibility to our patients to look after their health, as detailed in the NMC Code of Conduct (NMC, 2008), and this includes ensuring that their physical health needs are looked after. As we will see later in this chapter, physical activity plays a vital role in maintaining both mental and physical well-being. We also have a responsibility to provide a range of evidence-based interventions designed to improve outcomes for our patients, and as their advocates we should be looking at a range of options that allow our patients to become partners in care, but also equip them with skills to be able to manage their illnesses with more than medication alone.

So what are the benefits of physical activity?

Physical inactivity is the fourth leading risk factor for global mortality, and accounts for 6 per cent of deaths globally (World Health Organisation, WHO, 2010; DH, 2011b). Regular physical activity has a positive role to play in well-being, and can help prevent and manage over 20 chronic conditions, including coronary heart disease, stroke, type 2 diabetes, cancer, obesity, mental health problems and musculoskeletal conditions (WHO, 2010; DH, 2011b). This can then be translated into actual financial costs, which equate to approximately £1.06 billion and relate only to the cost of treating the five conditions directly related to physical inactivity (coronary heart disease, stroke, diabetes, colorectal cancer and breast cancer, DH, 2011b). It therefore is at best a conservative estimate as other conditions and diseases are not included. It also has a societal effect in terms of working days lost through sickness and premature death of people of working age. The benefits therefore apply both to individual physical and mental well-being, and to our wider society and economy.

How does it work?

Physical activity works as a stimulator to the body, putting stress on the cardiovascular, metabolic and musculoskeletal system and subsequently forcing the body to adapt to these changes. Adaption to this increased stress leads to the systems becoming more efficient and therefore healthier because of the nature of homeostasis that is found in humans. The mere act of activity also uses energy at a higher rate than sedentary behaviour, and as such enables the body to burn more of the energy stored in our food, so if this energy expenditure is at a higher rate than the energy consumption then weight loss should result (DH, 2011b).

The mechanism behind the benefits is felt to be two-fold, biochemical and psychological. Biochemically the action can be through the release of serotonin and endorphins and through altered stress reactivity and the adrenal/cortisol release. On a psychological level the action can have multifactorial benefits, for example through changes in body image and beliefs, health attitudes and beliefs, social reinforcement, increased mastery and improved coping skills.

Activity 6.2   *Reflection*

Think about the last time you were physically active. What impact did it have on your mental state both during and after?

Compare your findings to the evidence below.

Mental health benefits: the evidence

As nurses we see many patients suffering from anxiety disorders. There is now good evidence that physical activity can be as effective as cognitive behavioural therapy (CBT) with both acute and chronic anxiety, and more effective than other anxiety-reducing activities (Wipfli et al., 2008). Physical activity appears to benefit other groups of patients as well.

Panic disorder

In panic disorder physical activity can be considered to replicate exposure therapy with the similarity of physical activity symptoms to panic symptoms (DH, 2011b; Wolff et al., 2011).

Obsessive–compulsive disorder

With patients presenting with obsessive–compulsive disorder (OCD) the evidence indicates that physical activity combined with either pharmacological interventions or CBT reduces anxiety scores, with one study reporting acute reductions following 20- and 40-minute training sessions. However, these can only be considered as indicators due to small sample sizes and lack of control groups (DH, 2011b; Wolff et al., 2011).

Post-traumatic stress disorder

Post-traumatic stress disorder (PTSD) pilot studies suggest that physical activity has a positive effect on symptom severity; however the studies examined have methodological limitations and further research is needed in this area (DH, 2011b; Wolff et al., 2011).

Social phobia

At present there are no specific trials into the use of physical activity with social phobia, specific phobias or generalised anxiety disorders, but studies with mixed anxiety patients report larger reductions in anxiety, depression and stress in groups with CBT and physical activity as compared to CBT alone and other studies report that physical activity reduces anxiety sensitivity (DH, 2011b; Wolff et al., 2011).

Case study

Ella was referred by her GP to her local IAPT service with depression. She was keen to not take medication and wanted to try other treatments first. She had felt low in mood for a couple of years and could not identify any discernible cause for this. Her symptoms included feeling very low in energy with no motivation to do anything outside of work and feelings of hopelessness and disturbed sleep. Her practitioner suggested that she was experiencing temporary relief from avoiding anything outside of the basic necessities but that this was then making her feel worse as she did not experience any feelings of achievement. He suggested that behavioural activation would help and that some physical activity would fit this and hopefully improve her sleep. They negotiated re-introducing her trips to the local gym, which she had let slide over the last few months, starting with just one visit and increasing this as she felt some benefit. Over a period of six weeks she increased this to three visits a week and reported feeling much better both physically and mentally and that her sleep had begun to improve. She had also signed up for one of the gym's social events, and whilst slightly anxious about this was looking forward to seeing some of her old gym friends. She was discharged from the service and at a three-month follow up reported low scores on the PHQ9 and said that she had now added swimming to her gym visits and that her sleep had returned to normal.

The use of physical activity in affective disorders has a broader evidence base, showing significant benefits when used in conjunction with other treatments and as a stand-alone. A recent major depressive disorder meta-analysis found large clinical effects for physical activity alone with moderate effects in the long term. When compared to both pharmacology and CBT it was found to be as effective, and general physical activity at or above the public health recommended dose seemed more effective than lower intensities. In acute symptomology of depression physical activity has been found to increase positive mood and vigour when compared to quiet rest. However there were no statistically significant differences in distress, depression, confusion, fatigue, tension or anger. When considering longer-term responses, which are necessary due to the likelihood of relapse with major depressive disorders, physical activity had lower relapse rates than sertraline treatment alone. There is limited research when looking at physical activity and post-natal depression, however the current indications are that physical activity has a positive effect on depressive symptoms when compared to no physical activity. With bipolar disorder, where physical health comorbidity is prevalent, recent studies indicate a decrease in symptoms of stress, depression and anxiety, with increases in self-reported well-being. Further caution should be exercised here due to possible induction of manic episodes, and the fact that these studies are generally underpowered in terms of statistical significance (Wolff et al., 2011; DH, 2011b).

In patients with eating disorders, using physical activity is controversial because of the potential overuse of physical activity by patients with these problems. With binge eating disorder, where often patients are not physically active, studies report reductions in weight and BMI and depressive symptoms when used individually and with CBT. This was despite poor physical activity compliance both during and after treatment, which seems to support the psychological benefits of physical activity. With bulimia nervosa the research is limited but one study indicates that physical activity was as effective, or more effective than CBT depending on the outcome measurements used. Anorexia nervosa is a condition also limited in terms of statistically significant research, but the available evidence implies that light to moderate physical activity can have positive effects on attitudes and beliefs around physical activity, reductions in stress, protecting of bone mass and enhancing weight gain. Another study found neither benefit nor detrimental effects (Wolff et al., 2011).

In substance use disorders despite the number of studies the evidence can only be considered limited because of methodological factors. In smoking cessation, where the evidence is more robust, when physical activity is started prior to cessation with higher intensities (that is exercising at a higher heart rate, such as cycling above 14mph or including some periods of sprinting into a run) it is beneficial as a coping strategy, which regulates mood and reduces cravings. With alcohol and drugs, despite the methodological limitations, the evidence points to improved abstinence and reduced depressive and anxiety symptoms (Wolff et al., 2011).

Case study

John had smoked at least 20 cigarettes a day since he was 16 and decided that he wanted to give up at the age of 36. He had, like many smokers, attempted to give up in the past, with limited success. This time with the advice of the smoking cessation service he decided to use physical activity as the intervention and go 'cold-turkey'. He bought a bicycle and started to cycle a few weeks before he gave up smoking. On giving up smoking cycling started to have both a physiological effect as well as a psychological benefit. 'I would only allow myself to go out on my bicycle when I had not smoked the day before, and as I really enjoyed the cycle rides this soon became a stronger drive. Alongside of this I soon realised that to be able to go out on my bicycle more often and for longer distances having multiple days of not smoking increased

> *my endurance. It was then not long before the feeling I got after a bicycle ride, both emotionally and physically, outweighed the desire to have a cigarette'. John has continued to use this strategy and six years later has not smoked a cigarette since giving up.*

Psychotic illnesses present a challenge due to the nature and course of the illness. However recent randomised controlled trials (RCTs) found reductions in body fat, BMI and positive and negative symptoms and increases in functional capacity and quality of life when compared to standard care alone (Wolff et al., 2011).

The evidence with regards to mental health is therefore limited, except in the case of major depressive disorder, but you should consider this in the context of the limited research that is available, which has methodological complications.

Physical health benefits

By far the majority of research into the health benefits of physical activity acknowledges the benefit on mortality from all causes; current DH research indicates strong evidence and up to a 30 per cent reduction in risk of chronic disease. This is important information which you need to have to hand when talking to patients about the benefits of physical exercise.

Cardiovascular disease and the benefits of physical activity have been established for many years from the seminal work of Morris and Crawford (1958) who compared the mortality of bus drivers and conductors in the 1950s, and concluded that those in more physically active jobs were less likely to die prematurely from heart disease. This research has been built upon with prospective follow-up studies involving both men and women, some studies returning up to a 50 per cent reduction of risk from cardiovascular disease (DH, 2011b; Blair and Morris, 2009; Warburton et al., 2006) with some studies also finding evidence that there is a lower risk of premature death for those with risk factors for cardiovascular disease but who engage in regular activity than those with no risk factors but who lead a sedentary lifestyle (Warburton et al., 2006). The Warburton et al. (2006) review also identified positive benefits even for those with established cardiovascular disease, within limits, which are currently advised to be at intensity not in excess of 45 per cent of maximum heart rate, where maximum heart rate is the maximum rate the heart can sustain during very intense exercise, for up to a couple of minutes before exhaustion sets in.

An increase in type 2 diabetes risk is an increasing concern for many mental health patients as a result of lifestyle choices (and possibly some prescribed mental health medications (Disability Rights Commission, DRC, 2006)), however some reductions in this risk have been associated with regular physical activity; in one study a 6 per cent reduction in relative risk was associated with each energy expenditure of 500 kcal a week. In other words, patients are reducing their risk of type 2 diabetes with just one session a week, such as a brisk walk or an hour's swim. Warburton et al. (2006) found in a review of RCTs that modest weight loss through diet and exercise reduced the incidence of the disease among high risk people by 40–60 per cent over 3–4 years and the DH (2011b) identify a 30–40 per cent lower risk in moderately active people compared to those who are sedentary. Secondary protection for those with diabetes from physical activity reduced the incidence of all-cause premature death by 39–53 per cent (Orozco et al., 2008).

Case study

Joan was referred to a healthy living group at her local CMHT on diagnosis of type 2 diabetes alongside of her diagnosis of schizophrenia and was keen to avoid having to take extra medication on top of her antipsychotic medication. Her GP had agreed that she should try to control it through lifestyle, however prescribed her metformin in case this was not successful. She engaged very well in the healthy living group. It was run every two weeks with ten different topics covered each session, and the cycle was repeated at the end of week 10 and participants were able to dip in or out at any stage and could continue as long as they wished. Her main goals were those of lifestyle-controlled diabetes and a healthy lifestyle for her son and daughter who lived with her. She was a regular attendee at the group and was always an active participant both in the discussions and the weight measurement (which was voluntary), keen to learn both from the facilitators and other group members. She replaced all the sugary snacks in her house with fresh fruit, cooked a healthy meal every day (as opposed to ready meals) and started to walk to all of her appointments. At first this was difficult and her son and daughter offered much resistance, but with the support of the group she persisted and at her six-month review with her GP her BM measurements had returned to normal and her BMI was on its way down, and he agreed that she no longer needed the metformin prescription. She continued to attend the group after this and became a central figure offering support and guidance to new members but more importantly demonstrated to herself that she could positively improve her life without relying on medication. Whilst she was stable on her antipsychotic medication she reported fewer negative symptoms and felt that she now had some positive distractions when her voices grew worse.

Cancer prevention is associated with regular physical activity, particularly colon and breast cancer, where the reduction in risk has been estimated at 30–40 and 20–30 per cent, respectively (DH, 2011b; Warburton et al., 2006). The dose–response relationship is evident here with a greater protective effect of moderate intensity or above. It is felt that the benefit of physical activity will be conveyed to patients with current cancer, although there is a lack of research in this area. Qualitative research into the lived experience demonstrates that cancer sufferers report increases in quality of life with regular physical activity, however we are not clear about the precise role of physical activity here.

The impact that physical activity has on musculoskeletal health returns mixed results which are dependent on the type and frequency of activity. The DH (2011b) identifies evidence of moderate strength for bone health, particularly around hip and vertebral fractures and bone density. They report risk in reduction of 36–68 per cent at the highest levels of physical activity, whereas the magnitude of the effect of physical activity on bone mineral density is 1–2 per cent. Warburton et al. rightly identify that the type of activity can be crucial here; low impact activity has less of an effect than high impact. For early postmenopausal women and older women (75–85) studies demonstrate that intensive training involving either resistance or agility exercises are superior to stretching alone. With regards to joint health, the evidence is weak, but moderate-level activity does not lead to development of osteoarthritis unless there is major joint injury. There is strong evidence in support of physical activity for increasing skeletal muscle, however this is highly variable and dose dependent (DH, 2011b). There may be indications here for more research into elderly populations, as with increasing age aerobic activities become more prohibitive and resistance exercise may be a way of improving health outcomes, but also in improving or maintaining levels of independent living (Warburton et al., 2006).

So the evidence for positive effects on physical health is very strong, and whilst there is some evidence for a positive impact on mental health problems it is not so clear. Part of this may be due to the paucity of research into the specific effect of activity and the dose–response level, but it may also be due to the difficulty in measuring quality of life indicators as opposed to distinct biological markers. Studies into biological markers have identified a wealth of specific benefits and markers: weight control, enhanced lipid profiles, glucose homeostasis, reductions in blood pressure, reductions in systemic inflammation, improved blood circulation and cardiac function and enhanced endothelial function (DH, 2011b; WHO, 2010; Warburton et al., 2006). Psychologically the mechanisms of action are more subjective, but nevertheless just as important and include reductions in stress, anxiety and depression as well as feelings of self-esteem, mastery and accomplishment and routine activity scheduling. The fact is that at varying levels physical activity is going to positively improve the lives of our patients, but the question is how do we motivate and support them and how much should they do?

Recommended levels of activity

Activity 6.3 — *Reflection*

Make a note of how much activity you carried out over the past week and its intensity level. Note the type of activity, e.g. cycling, running, and how hard it felt: were you out of breath, or could you hold a conversation? Was this difficult?

Compare your notes with the recommended amounts of time and dose as outlined below.

Many of us exercise at very different levels or intensities and for differing amounts of time and it is therefore difficult to recommend a completely individualised amount and type of exercise. We must also not forget to include our job and transport to work: for example someone who cycles to work may see it as transport and not necessarily exercise; also a labourer on a building site is likely to have higher activity levels than an office worker.

The UK government has set out some clear guidelines for recommended activity, which are also internationally recommended by the World Health Organisation (DH, 2011b; WHO, 2010) (see Figure 6.1).

Early years (under 5s)	Children and young people (5–18)
Physical activity should be encouraged from birth and pre-school children who can walk unaided should be physically active for at least 180 minutes a day, with a minimal amount of time sedentary.	Moderate to vigorous intensity physical activity for at least 60 minutes and up to several hours each day. Vigorous intensity activities including activities that strengthen muscle and bone should be incorporated at least three days a week. Time spent being sedentary should be minimised.
Adults (19–64)	Older adults (65+)
Should aim to be active daily, and over a week this activity should add up to at least 150 minutes of moderate intensity activity carried out in bouts of at least 10 minutes or more. Comparable benefits can be achieved through 75 minutes of vigorous intensity activity spread across the week. Physical activity to improve muscle strength should be undertaken on at least two days a week and the time spent being sedentary should also be minimised.	All older adults should aim to be physically active as even some is better than none, ideally 150 minutes a week, in bouts of no less than 10 minutes should be achieved. For those regularly active at a moderate intensity comparable benefits can be gained through 75 minutes of vigorous intensity spread across the week, or a combination of moderate and vigorous activity. Physical activity that improves muscle strength should be undertaken on at least two days a week and older adults at risk of falls should undertake activity to improve balance and co-ordination at least two days a week. The time spent being sedentary should also be minimised.

Figure 6.1: Government recommendations for physical activity

Physical activity can be gained in various ways, through everyday activities such as cycling or walking to school or work, housework, gardening, DIY or occupational activity, active recreation and also through sport. Sedentary behaviours are multi-faceted and could include watching TV, using a computer, travelling by car, bus or train and sitting to read, talk or listen to music (DH, 2011b).

Concept summary: MET and RPE

Physically activity is scientifically expressed in METs (metabolic equivalent of task) where 1 MET is equal to sedentary energy expenditure, e.g. sitting quietly, therefore moderate intensity is characterised by 3–6 METs and vigorous intensity is characterised by greater than 6 METs. This, however, is not a user-friendly method of assessing our levels of physical activity. O'Donovan et al. (2010) and DH (2011b) suggest that practical measures to use are either ratings of perceived exertion (RPE), which uses a rating scale from 6 to 20, where 20 is maximum intensity which is sustainable only for a very short period of time and is very tiring, for example sprinting as hard as possible, and 6 is no exertion at all. Six may seem an odd starting point but it relates to heart rate, in that multiplying the RPE by 10 gives an approximate heart rate, and therefore moderate intensity would be 12–14 on the RPE scale. Alternatively we can use the 'talk test', whereby the ability to hold a light conversation roughly equates to moderate intensity, and difficulty maintaining any conversation equates to vigorous intensity. Clearly these measures are subjective, but they are much more user-friendly than METs and can be very accurate when compared to heart rates.

The DH (2011b) estimates that across the UK approximately 38 per cent of men and 28 per cent of women meet the minimum recommended levels of activity of 30 minutes of moderate intensity on at least five days a week. This is likely to be an over-estimate as most people exaggerate the amount of physical activity in self-reported surveys, and recent objective measures suggest significantly lower levels of participation of 6 per cent of men and 4 per cent of women in England according to accelerometer data (DH, 2011b). Health inequalities also negatively impact on this and can include income, gender, age, ethnicity and disability. The risks of taking part in physical activity are low, and those who are inactive are advised to gradually increase their activity. None the less anybody who is worried or concerned or has physical or mental health problems are advised to seek advice from their GP prior to starting to increase activity levels.

It is not possible here to give definitive outlines of exercises for our patients, but we can suggest some examples of applications to those suffering with mental health problems.

Depressed patients often avoid much activity, including physical activity, and encouraging them to take some walks, for example to their appointment with you, or during a keyworker session or as part of their leave entitlement can positively impact on their mood, as we saw in Ella's case study.

Starting a football group, both on an inpatient ward or as part of a community team can give some focus to a patient's day and increase their social contact as well as burning off some energy.

Setting up a garden project, through either the allotments of the local council or using your organisation's land gives a good dose of physical activity but also increases social contact and may even produce fruit or vegetables that your patients could enjoy!

So now we believe in physical activity and we understand what constitutes activity how do we promote, encourage and support our patients to build to and maintain this win–win strategy?

Activity 6.4   *Critical thinking*

Draw up a list of barriers that you experience when trying to engage in physical activity. How easy do you find it to overcome these? What barriers do you think patients may have to overcome?

Outline answers are given at the end of the chapter.

Cognitive interventions to promote and support patients

Before we push our patients out of the door to go for a run it is important that we are able to prepare them for the physical activity that they are going to engage in. This means that we have discussions with them to ascertain what they have done in the past, what they have enjoyed and what activity suits them best. As a clinician you may wish for the activity to have a distinct thera-peutic intervention, for example a patient with social phobia working towards joining a badminton group, however this must be a collaborative process. The use of a training plan, schedule or diary allows both the current level of activity to be measured while also scheduling new sessions or activities. Training schedules can be used alongside specific physical activity tools, such as heart rate monitors, however the most important element of the schedule or diary is that it is specific and the patient leaves the session knowing 'what, when, where and with whom'. The final element of our patient's preparation is that we need to discuss the barriers that may come between them and their chosen physical activity. You saw in Activity 6.4 that we all have barriers to engaging in physical activity but that we are more likely to overcome them if they form part of the plans and preparation to use this intervention.

It is important that physical activity remains fun and this means understanding your patient so you can help them to find the right physical activity for them. There are physical activities out there to suit everyone, ranging from national cycle routes to the more obscure, such as 'Run for Your Lives' where runners combine a 5k run with escaping from zombies! (See Sustrans and Run for Your Lives in Useful websites.) Planning some of the activities can be fun, and entering events allows a distinct goal to be set, and therefore the stages in achieving that goal. Keeping it fun allows numerous opportunities, for example bringing together five friends or patients to form a 5-a-side team, or antenatal aerobics, and this retains the social element, which exists beyond the physical activity alone. Your patients may want to involve the whole family and again there are numerous activities which a family can engage in with the advantage of the increased motivation that comes from a family activity, and also the positive benefit to all (see Change4Life in Useful websites).

Addressing the barriers

Finding the time to exercise is a barrier that often crops up; but it is very rarely a time issue and more of a priority management issue. The minimum activity levels (DH, 2011b) should be straightforward to implement into even the busiest of diaries when it is thought of as another schedule. To put this into context here in the UK we are the top nation for TV viewing and watch a staggering average of four hours a day.

The key to overcoming this issue is with SMART goals and scheduling. It helps if the goals are linked to the activity in some form and that you as clinician follow up regularly on the activity: its benefits, its barriers and achieving goals. This can be achieved through the use of an activity schedule to plan the activities, which then becomes a discussion point for the next therapy session where activity is reviewed in terms of values and goals.

Where is your gym bag, where are your walking shoes? Placing equipment and clothing in places where they are likely to be seen and ensuring that they are clean can help to trigger cognitive cues to be active, or to remember the feelings that are generated post-activity. Choosing the right clothes is very important as dressing the part can go a long way to improving motivation through factors such as adopting the role of the exerciser, therefore looking the part. Buying the right clothing can also be a motivational tool, for example buying a rain jacket for running in the rain can help motivate when the weather is bad, but it also can function as a reward. Appropriate clothing also ensures that you are comfortable during the physical activity.

Motivation

It is very important that we understand our patients' motivation to be active. Motivation can come from many sources, and can at times be unhelpful, for example motivation for activity that is based on outcomes can be difficult to maintain. I may wish to look like a TV soap life-saver, but if it is an unrealistic goal I will lose motivation when the rewards do not come quickly. We must as clinicians try to help our patients to focus on more tangible benefits such as the motivation for the process, or the effort that is required to get there. For example a patient with depression may find it hard to see how their goal of being physically active may help the depression, but they will experience a sense of mastery in achieving the three scheduled activities planned for the week, which then fuels the additional motivation to continue to use physical activity.

Motivation is not a fixed entity, but susceptible to change. We first need to be aware of the factors that impact on our ability to be motivated. Try drawing a hierarchy of competing motivations to help contextualise the barriers. For example watching TV may be the top of the hierarchy and going for that walk bottom; understanding this allows for the activity to be correctly scheduled so that the competing demands and desires are minimised. Have a walk now, watch your favourite TV show after. Think of motivation as a muscle: the more it is used the bigger and stronger the muscle becomes. Like a muscle it is influenced by fatigue and stress, which will ultimately lead to it becoming stronger and more resistant to the barriers and allow for successful planning of activities.

'Chaining' is a useful process that allows the motivation muscle to be stretched; it links little activities that lead to the ultimate goal. In discussion with your patient explore the last time they were, or tried to be, physically active. This analysis can lead to the construction of a number of small efforts that ultimately lead to being active. A possible example of this is given in Figure 6.2.

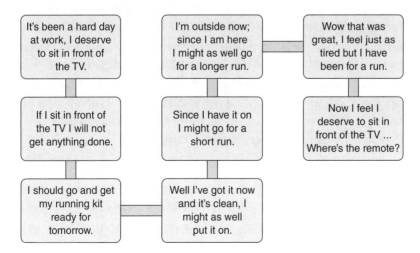

Figure 6.2: An example of the chaining process

By breaking up the task into specific smaller goals it makes the process less daunting for our patients. Once outside and running to the end of the street they are more likely to turn it into a half-hour run than they would be if they were at home on the sofa. This is not easy, but close exploration of the factors at play before activity can help to minimise the barriers. For example, our depressed patient sitting on the sofa may find the thought of going for a run impossible, but getting up and off the sofa is significantly more achievable. Exploring this with your patient may help you develop support tools, for example flash cards or motivational statements posted around the house. It also allows for other factors to be integrated such as having the gym kit ready, meeting with friends for that walk or choosing the best time to go for a cycle when there is less traffic on the roads.

Activity 6.5   *Decision making*

Using the model described, try devising chaining for some aspect of physical activity that you find difficult.

Compare how you felt before this exercise to how you feel after.

Attending to the negative thoughts

As identified in a previous chapter we all experience negative thoughts that impact on our ability and desire to do things. It is no different when looking at physical activity and subsequently the tools we use to overcome, or adapt to, these negative thoughts is similar.

The first stage is to identify the common thoughts that occur prior to activity, which can be achieved through exploration of a recent situation where your patient was, or was not, physically active. If physical activity has not been a feature of their lifestyle, imagining that they are about to be physically active can help to generate these negative thoughts. You can then objectively assess these thoughts and construct a revised or adaptive thought. An example of this could be the patient who says 'I am too tired to exercise' because of poor sleep; the revised thought after reviewing the evidence could be 'I sleep better after exercise'. We, and our patients, often use the word 'or' when we should in fact be using 'and'. Changing our language to ensure that 'or' is replaced with 'and' can also help shift a change in motivation, for example 'I can go for a run or I can sit and watch TV', where the revised statement could be 'I can go for a run and after I can sit and watch TV'. This revised statement allows for both activities to be performed, and the sitting down to watch TV also then functions as a reward.

Negative thoughts may also occur during the activity and it is important that we prepare our patients for the potential impact of these. The intensity of the activity may lead to negative thoughts such as when higher intensity activity increases our awareness of our bodily sensations, our increased heart rate may feel like we are going to have a heart attack. It is important to explore these feelings with your patients as it may be that the intensity is too high and that they need to reduce it to a more manageable level and thereby reduce over-exertion. There is a role for education and normalisation here as these symptoms are present for everyone and the biological responses to increased activity are also the same for all of us.

When considering the negative thought processes that may exist it is also worth bearing in mind the ones that can be generated as a result of the activity. These also need to be examined, for example, perfectionist tendencies, achieving that 'perfect' workout or attributing the aching or tiredness to mental or physical health symptoms rather than a direct result of the activity itself.

Enhancing the positives

Activity should be fun! Volkswagen converted a subway staircase into a piano keyboard, and discovered that 66 per cent of people used the stairs as opposed to the escalator (see Useful websites).

Mindfulness can be used to make exercise more interesting by helping us remain aware of the feelings of exercise, thereby attending to the physical sensations that are present during activity, and may mimic other physical sensations that may be present during day-to-day life. This therefore builds the awareness and skills of our patients to tolerate what are at times uncomfortable symptoms. Mindfulness may also be used to become more aware in general, by focusing on the environment in which the physical activity is being conducted, for example the breeze on the skin, or the colours of the leaves.

Finishing the activity on a high point can be very beneficial in the early stages of physical activity as we often only remember the latter stages of the activity, thereby 'finishing well' can have a positive memory boost for the next time.

It is important to construct some positive cycles of thought after the activity. The first of these is simply acknowledging what you have done and simple affirmation statements ('That was great! Didn't I do well?') can greatly assist in the process. These can be discussed prior to the activity, for example imagining how you might feel after that one-hour walk, writing these down and then adding the thoughts and feelings that occur after the exercise. One of the most efficient ways of doing this is through the use of a diary, which can be subjective for your patients, but could include mood ratings before and after the activity or be as complex as the patient chooses. A positive cognitive cycle can then be developed linking activity to mood improvements which then leads to increased motivation to be more active, which then feeds into being more active. This positive cycle can be shown next to a traditional negative one (see Figure 6.3), such as avoiding activity leads to feelings of relief, which are quickly replaced by feelings of guilt and shame, thereby reducing motivation to be active and the result being a reduction in activity. These cycles help your patients in times of low motivation to be physically active.

Making activity part of our daily lives again can assist in this process. At the beginning of the chapter we saw how underactive we are compared to our forebears. We need to make activity a normal part of day-to-day life. This can be simple, such as playing with the children, going for walks with friends or family, even using the stairs as opposed to lifts or escalators. Even on a most basic level this is important; the DH (2011b) identified that sedentary behaviour is on its own a significant risk factor for chronic illnesses and thereby reducing this increases the quality and longevity of life for all people.

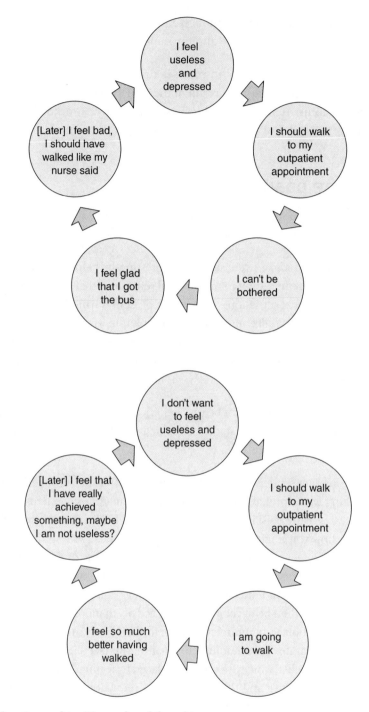

Figure 6.3: Negative and positive cycles of thought

Some cautions

There are very few cautions with physical activity; as identified in much of the literature it is a 'win–win' situation with both physical and mental health benefits. The most significant caution is to ensure that your patient is physically able to be active, which would include a discussion with the GP or the consultant in charge of the patient's care prior to engaging in a physical activity programme. In any case, it is important to start gently and build up the activity gently over time.

Eating disorders (ED) are the one disorder where physical activity should be used very carefully because it can be a strategy to lose weight, or create an ideal body image. This is not helped with some of the media images and stereotypes of athletes. Physical activity can be both addictive and a distraction for those with EDs and as such should be discussed in much more depth with the care team. Physical activity can be very beneficial for those with ED, but should be used with a degree of objectivity and control.

Chapter summary

We have considered the evidence for physical activity here, both with mental health and physical health problems. Whilst there is much stronger evidence for the use of physical activity in the physically unwell there are clear benefits to those suffering with mental illness. This could be as a result of different markers for the success of physical activity, or the lack of research into mental health benefits. There are clear national and international guidelines for levels of activity, which are linked to a dose response. Finally we have considered some of the barriers that may arise in both the planning and implementation of physical activity as an intervention and looked at therapeutic ways to overcome these barriers.

Activities: brief outline answers

Activity 6.4 Critical thinking

Barriers can be very personal and as such we must respect this. For example the socially anxious patient may find any social situation terrifying which may be at odds to our beliefs. Some common examples of barriers include:

- lack of time;
- medication;
- no one to exercise with;
- financial constraints;
- my illness stops me;
- what if I feel worse?
- the weather.

How do these compare to your lists?

Further reading

Biddle, SJH, Fox, KR and Boutcher, SH (eds) (2000) *Physical Activity and Psychological Well-Being*. London: Routledge.
Slightly more emphasis on exercise and mental health, and again a useful text on the positive use of physical activity for psychological disorders.

Department of Health (DH) (2011) *Start Active, Stay Active: A report on physical activity from the four home countries' Chief Medical Officers.* London: Stationery Office.
An insight into how physically inactive we are as a nation here in the UK.

Faulkner, G and Taylor, A (eds) (2005) *Exercise, Health and Mental Health: Emerging Relationships.* London: Routledge.
This is a useful book which looks at the relationship between exercise and general and mental health.

Useful websites

www.change4life.icnetwork.co.uk
Change for Life is a UK government initiative to increase healthy lifestyles through activity and healthy eating. It is a useful website as it has helpful tips, facts and suggestions.

www.creativity-online.com/work/volkswagen-fun-theory-piano-staircase/17522
Piano staircase, an initiative by Volkswagen to increase the use of stairs as opposed to escalators.

www.nationmaster.com/graph/med_tel_vie-media-television-viewing
TV watching league tables.

www.runforyourlives.com
Run for Your Lives (the zombie run) is a fun run aimed at encouraging people into activity through new and novel ways. This one combines a run with trying to evade the zombie hordes!

www.sustrans.co.uk
Sustrans is a national charity which campaigns for healthy options to enable people to travel to work, school and other activities by foot, cycles and public transport. They operate a series of national cycle paths.

Chapter 7
Dual diagnosis

Kim Moore

NMC Standards for Pre-registration Nursing Education

This chapter will address the following competencies:

Domain 1: Professional values
All nurses must act first and foremost to care for and safeguard the public. They must practise autonomously and be responsible and accountable for safe, compassionate, person-centred, evidence-based nursing that respects and maintains dignity and human rights. They must show professionalism and integrity and work within recognised professional, ethical and legal frameworks. They must work in partnership with other health and social care professionals and agencies, service users, their carers and families in all settings, including the community, ensuring that decisions about care are shared.

2.2.1   Mental health nurses must practise in a way that addresses the potential power imbalances between professionals and people experiencing mental health problems, including situations when compulsory measures are used, by helping people exercise their rights, upholding safeguards and ensuring minimal restrictions on their lives. They must have an in-depth understanding of mental health legislation and how it relates to care and treatment of people with mental health problems.

4.4   All nurses must be self-aware and recognise how their own values, principles and assumptions may affect their practice. They must maintain their own personal and professional development, learning from experience, through supervision, feedback, reflection and evaluation.

4.41   Mental health nurses must actively promote and participate in clinical supervision and reflection, within a values-based mental health framework, to explore how their values, beliefs and emotions affect their leadership, management and practice.

NMC Essential Skills Clusters (ESCs)

This chapter will address the following ESCs:

6.   People can trust the newly registered graduate nurse to engage therapeutically and actively listen to their needs and concerns, responding using skills that are helpful, providing information that is clear, accurate, meaningful and free from jargon.

(continued)

continued ...

> 6.8 Communicates effectively and sensitively in different settings, using a range of methods and skills.
>
> 6.12 Uses the skills of active listening, questioning, paraphrasing and reflection to support a therapeutic intervention.
>
> 9. People can trust the newly registered graduate nurse to treat them as partners and work with them to make a holistic and systematic assessment of their needs; to develop a personalised plan that is based on mutual understanding and respect for their individual situation promoting health and well-being, minimising risk of harm and promoting their safety at all times.
>
>> 9.16 Promotes health and well-being, self-care and independence by teaching and empowering people and carers to make choices in coping with the effects of treatment and the ongoing nature and likely consequences of a condition including death and dying.
>>
>> 9.18 Discusses sensitive issues in relation to public health and provides appropriate advice and guidance to individuals, communities and populations for example, contraception, substance misuse, smoking, obesity.

Chapter aims

After reading this chapter you will be able to:

- describe the different expressions of dual diagnosis in all fields of nursing;
- understand common relationships between mental health and substance use;
- describe perceptions of the dual diagnosis patient group;
- understand some of the treatments available.

Introduction

As a student nurse you will experience many different placements across a variety of settings during your course, and no matter which branch of nursing you are working in, you are likely to have direct contact with a person experiencing a dual diagnosis, in this context meaning someone with mental health and substance abuse problems. If we are to act as advocates for the equality of all our patients, and work to challenge the stigma associated with mental health, then we must also challenge the stigma associated with dual diagnosis cases.

Drugs, alcohol and prescription drug use and misuse frequently occur in all health settings; in mental health services individuals with a dual diagnosis are viewed as 'an expectation rather than an exception' (Department of Health, DH, 2002; UK Gov, 2000). Nursing care of dual diagnosis patients can be confusing and difficult to understand, with diverse and competing health and social care issues (Waddell and Skäräter, 2007), treatment cultures and oppositional philosophies. Nurses are expected to engage and promote change with patients known to have increased symptom severity, increased risk of self-harm and violence towards others and have poor treatment compliance while working in collaboration with colleagues without a shared language or approach (Rassool, 2006). It is in this context that nurses working in dual diagnosis are faced with significant challenges that can leave them feeling disempowered and frustrated (NMC, 2002; Phillips, 2007). Despite this, all nurses (student or qualified) are expected to be proactive advocates for all their patients (NMC, 2008).

Nurses and nursing students have important roles in undertaking dual diagnosis assessment and interventions (Rassool and Rawaf, 2008; Tran et al., 2009; Lovi and Barr, 2009). The publication of *The Good Practice Guide: Dual Diagnosis* (DH, 2002) directed services and clinicians to provide therapeutic interventions at different stages, collaborating with diverse teams and services. It is no longer acceptable to dismiss the needs of the person as 'just a drug/alcohol problem' or 'too mad' to engage in treatment interventions. Mental health and substance misuse nurses may be the identified 'key' players (Edward and Munroe, 2009), however dual diagnosis patients will access acute care, child and adolescent services, maternity and prisons. This chapter aims to provide insight into the different expressions of dual diagnosis in all fields of nursing, examine some common relationships between mental health and substance use, explore perception of the dual diagnosis patient group and explore some of the treatment options that can be used in interacting with individuals who have a dual diagnosis.

Nursing and dual diagnosis

One of the principal values of nursing is to 'make the care of people your first concern treating them as individuals and respecting their dignity' (NMC, 2008, p3). In your placements you will undoubtedly come into contact with people who have mental health problems, drug or alcohol use and dual diagnosis. From maternity and paediatrics to older people you are likely to meet someone with a dual diagnosis; they may be a patient or a relative and you will need to be able to interact and act as an advocate on their behalf. As a student nurse you are unlikely to receive formal training on working with dual diagnosis patients, despite the known prevalence of the patient group and the knowledge of their increased risks of psychological disturbance, cardiac problems, diabetes and dental issues; nursing students within all branches of health will work with dual diagnosis patients in all domains of healthcare (Canaway and Merkes, 2010).

Defining dual diagnosis

Activity 7.1   *Reflection*

The term dual diagnosis was 'borrowed' from learning disabilities services and is used as a label when a person has two health conditions occurring at the same time.

1. What definition does the World Health Organisation use for dual diagnosis?
2. Do you find this definition of 'dual diagnosis' helpful or not – what is the evidence for your decision?

You may have found a number of different descriptions for dual diagnosis, such as co morbid, concurrent, co-occurring, complex need, substance misusing mental health or mental health substance using patient. The World Health Organisation defines dual diagnosis as 'referring to co morbidity or the co-occurrence in the same individual of a psychoactive substance use disorder and another psychiatric disorder' (WHO, 2014). Dual diagnosis is one of the more common terms used to describe this phenomenon, but you may also have found the term MICA (mentally ill chemically abusing) and CAMI (chemically abusing mentally ill).

Research on nursing attitudes towards dual diagnosis consistently illustrates that many nurses feel frustrated, resentful and powerless when faced with patients who have a dual diagnosis (Deans and Soar, 2005; Rassool et al., 2006; Brouselle et al., 2007). It is equally clear that improving nurses' knowledge and skills in dual diagnosis positively affects their level of confidence, improving professional judgements and attitudes (Edward and Robin, 2012; Tran et al., 2009; Rani and Byrne, 2012; McCabe et al., 2011).

As we saw earlier, we bring preconceived ideas to the nursing of dual diagnosis patients. In the next activity we start to examine our beliefs.

Activity 7.2   *Reflection*

Read the following statements and consider how strongly you agree or disagree with each one; use your first thought or strongest feeling.

Strongly agree   Agree   Disagree   Strongly disagree

- Older adults (over the age of 65) do not use drugs.
- Drug users are all selfish, and their problems are self-inflicted.
- Drug/alcohol use is a lifestyle choice.
- Mental health patients who use drugs/alcohol are dangerous and violent.
- It is unlikely that I would have to nurse a patient with a dual diagnosis.

There is no answer as such, but some outline guidance information is given at the end of the chapter.

Before 2002, mental health and addiction nurses gave little recognition to individuals who had mental health and substance misuse problems; it was someone else's problem. This led to individuals being refused services and treatment as 'ineligible'. Making assumptions about the 'primacy of the problem' can lead to the most visible symptoms being interpreted as the problem rather than underlying issues, e.g. mental or physical health problems, which may be influencing the substance misuse behaviour. This diagnostic overshadowing is used to validate services' refusal of treatment, legitimising their avoidance of the dual diagnosis patient group (Coombes and Wratten, 2007). Strong feelings were and continue frequently to be provoked with moral and ethical opinions leading to negative views of successful treatment or 'treatment pessimism' (Coombes and Wratten, 2007; Edward and Robin, 2012). Given these factors should we wonder why dual diagnosis patients are less likely to be compliant with treatment?

How might dual diagnosis present?

We might see patients who have developed dual diagnosis for a number of reasons. There are several possible causes identified in the *Dual Diagnosis Good Practice Guide* (DH, 2002, p7), including:

- a primary psychiatric illness precipitating or leading to substance misuse;
- a substance misuse worsening or altering the course of a psychiatric illness;
- intoxication and/or substance dependence leading to psychological symptoms;
- substance misuse and/or withdrawal leading to psychiatric symptoms or illness.

Dual diagnosis includes all mental health conditions, from anxiety and depression to psychosis and dementia, and people with these illnesses may simultaneously use any one of a wide range of substances – including alcohol, prescription medications, over-the-counter products, 'legal herbal highs' and illegal drugs. You might rightly think that the combinations of these two problems are infinite, and in one respect you are right – both are extensive topics and rarely does the individual have two clearly identified issues (Rassool, 2006). You will encounter mixed mental health presentations combined with polysubstance use and complicated by physical health problems and social needs (Tolliver, 2010), however, you will also meet individuals who have problematic or occasional substance use, with less severe mental health diagnoses.

Concept summary: The scale of the problem

The International Classification of Diseases (ICD) records 99 distinct mental disorders (WHO, 1992), while over 200 substances are registered under the Misuse of Drugs Act (United Kingdom Government, 1971). This is an inordinate amount of potential dual diagnosis combinations.

Mental health and addictions do share some common features. They have similar profiles with large numbers of people sharing one diagnosis like stress, depression and anxiety in mental health, and in addictions a greater number use substances like alcohol, cannabis and cocaine. At the other end of the spectrum are individuals with less frequent mental health diagnoses like body dysmorphic disorder and postnatal psychosis, while in addictions this relates to the use of methamphetamine, khat and LSD. A third dimension to be considered is that in both cases there is variance in the severity of the symptoms or the level of distress and symptomology in mental health and the dependency (amount and frequency) in addictions. However, as you can see, dual diagnosis has some overlap between mental health and addiction services, but does not fit neatly into any discipline (see Figure 7.1).

Developing therapeutic relationships is linked to how we use our interpersonal communication skills; there is no difference in developing these therapeutic alliances with people who experience either mental health or addictions issues. What is critical in all professional

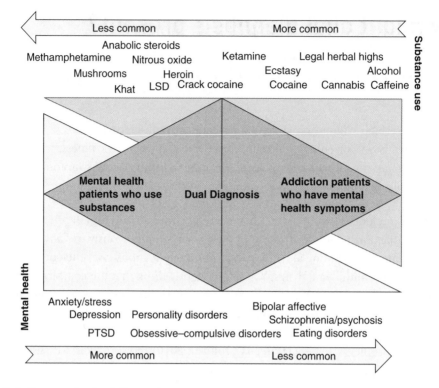

Figure 7.1: Patterns in dual diagnosis presentations

interactions is taking a non-judgemental approach and that you interact with the person, not their diagnosis or reputation. It is *your* knowledge and understanding of mental health and addiction problems and terminology that will enable you to make links and associations within individual cases, enabling informed discussion of their experience and potential treatment choices.

Activity 7.3   *Evidence-based practice and research*

Research the main drug effects in intoxication and withdrawal for all these substances:

Redbull	Cocaine	Khat	Ketamine
Alcohol	Heroin	Ecstasy	Solvents

Find out and note:

1. What category of drug do they belong to? (Stimulant, depressant, hallucinogenic or other.)
2. What are the main symptoms of intoxication?
3. What are the main symptoms of withdrawal?

Outline answers are provided at the end of the chapter.

Common dual diagnosis presentations

Your exploration of different drugs might have suggested that there are a number of similar symptoms shared by drug and alcohol intoxication and withdrawal states and mental health. Confusion can occur not only in relation to effects of combined drug, alcohol and mental health issues, but in the knowledge that some of these drug types, such as stimulants and opiates, are used in the treatment of physical and mental health conditions. Understanding the theory of how different illicit drugs and alcohol affects our psychology is helpful, and linking this to mental health presentations extends our understanding; however the experience of interacting with dual diagnosis patients in real-life situations can vary dramatically.

Activity 7.4   *Reflection*

Can you think of a person with a dual diagnosis you have recently been in contact with as a student nurse?

- What are the clearest memories you have about this person? Are they positive or negative?
- Can you think of two things you may have learned from this person that affected how you might positively engage with another dual diagnosis patient in the future?

For many nurses, their memory of working with a person who has a dual diagnosis is negative, and earlier this was described as feelings of frustration, resentment and helplessness. Our memories are influenced by what we feel; we recall negative events more clearly than many others (Kensinger, 2007) but they are subject to distortions. It may have been easier to recall negative memories of interactions with dual diagnosis patients; identifying positive learning may take some deep reflection. Let's have a closer look at some of the common dual diagnosis presentations you are likely to encounter in clinical practice.

Alcohol

Of all the substances used or prescribed, alcohol is one of the most dangerous (Royal College of Psychiatrists, RCP, 2013); despite this many of us will drink alcohol socially. You may recall that alcohol acts as a depressant drug (Drinkaware, 2013), but did you know that in 2010, 68,825 adult hospital admissions linked to alcohol related disease were recorded in the UK (Harker, 2012)? The social impact of moderate alcohol use can impact on physical health, employment, finance and relationships, factors that are also common with many mental health conditions. Heavy or dependant drinking increases physical and psychological effects increasing the impact of symptom severity in anxiety, depression, suicidal thinking and psychosis (RCP, 2013; British Liver Trust, 2014).

The self-medication hypothesis links the use of the depressant effects of alcohol with the need to calm states of arousal like stress and anxiety, or in the belief that it improves low mood (RCP, 2014). Increasingly alcohol use is a feature in disorders such as self-management of childhood trauma (Tomlinson et al., 2006) and post-traumatic stress disorders (PTSD) (RCP, 2014; Kitchner et al., 2011). These effects are linked to chemical and electrical messaging in the brain affecting thoughts, feelings and behaviours (Bartsch et al., 2007). A small amount of alcohol reduces inhibition, thus increasing confidence, something that might appeal to a person who lacks confidence or is stressed, anxious or experiencing auditory perceptual disturbances. Increased alcohol use over longer periods of time has a direct proportional relationship to negative physical and psychological effects (Drinkaware, 2013). Alcohol withdrawal rebound is when the depressing/suppressing effects of alcohol wear off – you experience an over-production of glutamine (the body's natural stimulant) causing hangover effects like disrupted sleep, anxiety and increased blood pressure (Finn and Crabbe, 1997; Tomlison et al., 2006), including lowering the seizure threshold which is why you may see alcohol withdrawal seizures (NICE, 2014).

Cannabis

You may be aware that cannabis alters perceptions affecting all our senses (auditory, olfactory, visual and touch), but did you know that cannabis use is commonly associated with a range of mental health issues? There was a long held view that cannabis caused psychosis and schizophrenia (Stefanis et al., 2004), and it is now known that cannabis is one element associated with triggering vulnerabilities for schizophrenia (Parakh and Basu, 2013; Cohen et al., 2008). Cannabis use is also associated with anxiety disorders and obsessive–compulsive disorders (OCD) but Mancebo et al. (2009) highlight that juvenile onset of OCD is more likely to be associated with alcohol rather than cannabis use and suggest that receiving OCD treatment may in itself reduce substance use.

There is another side to the story. Did you know that cannabis has many supporters promoting legalisation for treatment and recreational use? There are claims that cannabis is beneficial as treatment for physical health problems including Tourette's syndrome (Muller-Vahl et al., 2003; Baker et al., 2003; Amer, 2006), epilepsy (NHS Choices, 2014; Amer, 2006), pain (Ware et al., 2010; Baker et al., 2003; Amer, 2006) and multiple sclerosis (Baker et al., 2003; Amer, 2006). The potential for use in the treatment for nausea, appetite stimulation, epilepsy and glaucoma is suggested by Amer (2006), however glaucoma treatment is not supported by the Glaucoma Research Foundation (2013, www.glaucoma.org). Some users promote cannabis as treatment for asthma; the New Zealand Asthma Foundation (2010) opposes this view, promoting the opinion that cannabis when smoked is more harmful than tobacco.

Psychiatrists are deeply divided in their views on prescription cannabis, however Kweskin (2013) suggests that in some cases prescription cannabis would be considered not only for physical symptoms, but for some mental health symptoms including PTSD, mania, anxiety and sleep. What may be more concerning to health professionals is the increasing use of synthetic cannabis products found within the legal herbal high markets; there is considerably less known about the medium- and longer-term effects of synthetic cannabis, particularly in relation to mental health well-being and psychosis (ECDMMA, 2011).

Stimulants and mood disorders

Do you need to have a cup of tea or coffee to wake you up and get you going in the morning? If this is you, then you are using stimulants to alter your level of consciousness. Most of us have some knowledge of the effects of stimulants; mainly on increasing wakefulness and mood – our use of caffeine. Stimulants are thought to increase dopamine levels in the brain (Nash, 1997) in a dose correlated relationship; the higher the dose the more intense the positive feelings like elation, euphoria and self-satisfaction, however there is an association for some individuals with stimulants and psychosis (Sara et al., 2013).

Stronger stimulants such as cocaine, khat and methamphetamine all have similar effects of level of consciousness and mood, but to different degrees of intensity, and are frequently associated with episodes of psychosis (Sara et al., 2013). However, cocaine use is also associated with a diagnosis of ADHD (Ohlmeier et al., 2008). You might rightly assume that stimulant drugs promote feelings of well-being, energy and euphoria which might be helpful for treatment of severe depression. Historically, psychostimulants were used in the treatment of fatigue and depression (Ng and O'Brien, 2009; Stotz et al., 1999) but this is no longer the case because of concerns about misuse and drug tolerance.

Within your own peer or age groups, you may be aware that recreational stimulant use (cocaine, amphetamine and crack cocaine) remains high; however in the UK, this pattern is changing and there are currently reducing trends in cocaine use that may be influenced by the rise in 'herbal highs' (European Monitoring Centre for Drugs and Drug Addiction, EMCDDA, 2012) including mephedrone. These have similar profiles for intoxication and withdrawal to other stimulants, but with extreme symptoms of paranoia, violent outbursts and reduced motor control (Winder et al., 2013).

What is clear is the depression of mood during the withdrawal phase is of equal intensity to the high; such mood swings can easily mimic rapid cycling mood disorders such as bipolar affective disorder. Physical problems are found in relation to stimulant use including accidental death; however the most commonly seen within A&E departments include tachycardia, cardiac arrhythmias, convulsions or disorientation and confusion (Sadler, 2006). Long-term risks include high blood pressure, cardiac events and strokes.

Prescription stimulants and alcohol

Attention deficit hyperactivity disorder is a diagnosis you may be familiar with; you may be aware this has been one of the fastest growing diagnoses in child and adolescent services for the past ten years. Standard treatment of the three core symptoms (hyperactivity, impulsivity and inattention) is prescription stimulants; however questions are being raised about this practice (Meaux et al., 2006). You might also be aware of using stimulants to improve memory, which has led to a growing 'black market' in prescription stimulants at universities and reported as endemic in student populations worldwide (Arria and DuPont, 2010).

Do alcohol use and ADHD occur together? Researchers began exploring this question and many found a higher than average use of alcohol and stimulant drugs (Ohlmeier et al., 2008). This view is support by Huntley et al. (2012), whose investigation of undiagnosed ADHD in UK alcohol detoxification centres found individuals with undiagnosed ADHD were more likely to have an alcohol dependency, or use cocaine and amphetamines. Both alcohol and stimulant use were linked to increased frequency of depression and suicide attempts in these groups.

Opiates

You might think that people with a diagnosis of personality disorder, and in particular borderline personality disorder (BPD), are more likely to use opiates or alcohol. Talimbekova and Nurkhodjaev (2010) suggest this diagnosis worsens the degree and progression rate of dependency, and severity of opiate withdrawal. A number of biological theories have been suggested for this association including a reduction in neuro-chemical sensitivity to opiates or an opiate deficient model (Bandelow et al., 2010; New and Stanley, 2010).

What you may not be aware of is the use of opiates in PTSD which is a growing area of investigation, partially due to prescription opiate use as pain control following physical trauma. Current research suggests that opiate use in PTSD creates emotional numbing, dampening the emotional confusion and importantly suppressing the key symptom of over arousal. These models suggest that opiate use in PTSD is critically linked to self-medication of anxiety based symptoms (Reddy et al., 2013).

Less common is the beneficial relationship between opiates and OCD suggested by Rojas-Corrales et al. (2007) including prescription Tramadol linked to positive symptom reduction in Tourette's syndrome. In the case of opiate use and depression, you may think that the dampening effects of opiates would trigger depression, yet stage three drug trials for a non-addictive opiate treatment for severe treatment-resistant depression are being undertaken and the action of the drug is based on modulation of the opioid system in the brain (Business Wire, 2014).

Case study

Ed is 27 years old. He has a diagnosis of schizophrenia and regularly uses alcohol and cannabis. Ed began to experience symptoms of schizophrenia at the age of 19; he has had one admission to a mental health unit under a section 2 of the Mental Health Act (1983) at the age of 22, but has been stable for some time and he engages with community support. Ed experiences auditory hallucinations: he hears his grandfather's voice which can be supportive or abusive to him. He has two children (aged 1 and 9 years old), from different relationships. In both cases the pregnancies were unplanned. While Ed was excited to become a father, he became overly protective of his partner and the baby; to manage these feelings Ed smoked cannabis to make himself feel calmer, and discovered alcohol would quiet any suspicious thoughts. As a consequence Ed's cannabis use increased to ¼ oz and one can of 6 per cent beer on a regular basis. He became increasingly suspicious resulting in each of his relationships breaking down, and Ed no longer has contact with his children.

Over the past two years, Ed has become increasingly isolated. He is now a heavy user of cannabis (¼ oz/day) and four cans of 8 per cent alcohol per day, using this to stop thinking and feeling he is a 'bad father'; he has tried to stop on a number of occasions, but without success. Ed is unaware of his level of paranoia or that he responds verbally to the voice in his head; he has not noticed that the voice is mainly derogatory. Ed is avoiding all family contact; he believes he is being talked about behind his back and that everyone is plotting against him. He has thoughts of ending his life, and has refused to talk about how he is feeling as he believes that if he does say he is depressed he will be taken to hospital against his will.

<table>
<tr><td>

Activity 7.5

</td><td>

Critical thinking

</td></tr>
</table>

- Read the case study again and identify Ed's key mental health and substance use symptoms. Would this be considered a 'dual diagnosis case'? Why is this?
- How might your perception of this case change if Ed was an older person with adult children, or a woman?

Outline answers are provided at the end of the chapter.

Dual diagnosis nursing: windows of opportunity

Dual diagnosis patients lead complicated lives, with a diverse range of physical, social and psychological needs for which we as nurses are often unprepared. Earlier we explored how working with dual diagnosis patients can provoke some strong feelings, moral and ethical opinions, and treatment pessimism (Coombes and Wratten, 2007; Edward and Robin, 2012). Traditional approaches to treatment have been ineffective in supporting dual diagnosis patients to access treatment and make changes (United Kingdom Drug Policy Commission, UKDPC, 2012), so a good place to start is developing questions or curiosity about the person you are screening, and using your interpersonal skills to probe these questions. To help you formulate a nursing assessment and interventions, let's revisit Ed's case. Ed is experiencing altered perceptions (voices and paranoia) and is using alcohol and cannabis. We can analyse the issues in Table 7.1.

Intervening in dual diagnosis

Many nurses express concern that they do not have the 'right knowledge' to work with dual diagnosis cases and you may feel this way yourself, however it is suggested that nurses not only have these skills but they are more likely to be in the right place with more opportunities to interact (Moore and Rassool, 2008; Tran et al., 2009; Lovi and Barr, 2009). Whether the contact you make is a brief 'one off' assessment, or an ongoing therapeutic relationship, there are several clinical approaches that you could use, including:

- interpersonal communication skills (Bach and Grant, 2009)
- harm minimisation strategies(British Medical Association, BMA, 2013)
- motivational interviewing(Miller and Rollnick, 2012)
- psycho-education (Anderson et al., 1981)
- transtheoretical change models (Prochaska and DiClemente, 1982).

One or all of these approaches can be used in a staged or stepped approach that maximises the use of limited resources. You need to match the needs of the patient to the right level of care as a starting point, then step up or down in skill or intensity as treatment outcomes are being achieved (Von Korff and Tiemens, 2000).

Key issues	Nursing assessment	Nursing considerations
Risk of self-harm/suicide	Ed has talked about ending his life – does he have a plan? Ed not only feels depressed but that he lacks in self-worth and feels hopeless. Ed might have unresolved grief/loss reaction in relation to his children that underpin these risks.	What knowledge does Ed have about low mood and alcohol affecting mood? How strong are Ed's feelings about suicide and do they increase with alcohol use? How does Ed feel when he reduces or stops either his cannabis or alcohol use? Ed might experience 'rebound' effects if he stops alcohol without support; this would increase the amount, duration and intensity of any negative thoughts and feelings. Ed could potentially be at a higher level of risk when addressing his cannabis and alcohol use.
Experiencing and responding to auditory hallucinations	Ed has been observed responding to unseen conversations.	Does the voice command him to act? What is the frequency and level of intensity of this voice? What helps to reduce the frequency and intensity of this voice and how long does this last? Are there any links to either cannabis or alcohol use? When did the voice go from being supportive to abusive? Are there any links to either cannabis or alcohol use?
Experience of paranoia leading to isolation from others	Ed is suspicious of others; he believes everyone is talking about him and plotting against him.	Develop a trust relationship with Ed. Involve Ed in conversations and decisions. Consider Ed as an expert in his own care. Short interventions as Ed will tolerate being with others. Work with Ed to develop his story and plan of care (personalise).

		What helps to reduce the frequency and intensity of the paranoia and how long does this last? Are there any links to either cannabis or alcohol use? What helps to reduce the frequency and intensity of this voice and how long does this last? Are there any links to either cannabis or alcohol use?
Ability to self-soothe	Ed's use of cannabis and alcohol as a calming agent.	What other strategies has Ed tried in the past to help calm himself? Explore with Ed self-soothing strategies including 'staying in the moment', distraction, stress management and relaxation. What are the positive effects for Ed when using: • cannabis • alcohol
Cannabis and alcohol use	The frequency, amount, and method of using: • cannabis • alcohol	What is Ed's understanding of how these drugs work – what is his experience? What is Ed's knowledge and experience of cutting down or stopping these drugs? What is Ed's knowledge on safe use of these drugs? Are there any links Ed has made between the drug use and his mental health? Are there any links Ed has made between the drug use and potential or actual physical health problems?

Table 7.1: Assessment of Ed's case

Concept summary

- Harm reduction (HR) strategies for addictions emerged in the UK following publication of the Rolleston committee recommendations in the 1920s, concluding that in some cases continued drug maintenance may be necessary to help drug users. The HR approach is based on principles of not changing the behaviour, but in making this behaviour safer.
- Motivational interviewing (MI) was developed using Rodgers' client-centred approaches primarily working to enhance 'talk of change' to assist developing new thoughts and behaviours that enable change.
- Psycho-education (PE) became popular in the early 1980s and is based on the premise that improving and supporting how individuals gain an understanding specific to their illness allows them to develop a resource of tools that improves their ability to manage their condition in the longer term.
- Change theory (CM) (trans-theoretical model) identifies discrete stages on how decisions for change are internally processed; this model is frequently used in addiction treatment in combination with MI strategies.

Treatment outcomes take time

Change is not easy; in dual diagnosis small incremental changes are considerable achievements. If you are expecting to see dramatic rapid changes you may be disappointed, which is one of the factors leading to our sense of frustration and hopelessness. In complex cases change happens over the long term; months not weeks, or years rather than months – but it can and does happen. In situations where the mental health or substance use is less intrusive, change can happen at a faster pace. For many cases, where the degree of mental distress or substance use is beginning to become problematic, taking a positive psycho-educational approach has the potential for significant change over a short period. Depending on the nursing role you are in you may be a witness to this change, or in many cases you may never know.

Scenario

Imagine you are nursing Ed, 27, who has schizophrenia, smokes cannabis and drinks alcohol. Ed's case is highly complex, but he may be open to change. Let's consider how we might use a variety of interventions to promote and support change (see Table 7.2).

But what happens if Ed is not ready to make any change? Let's assume that Ed is not willing to make changes in his cannabis use, but he has had a negative experience of alcohol and has already tried to change this. Knowing this could provide you with a window of opportunity to help Ed make changes to his use of alcohol (see Table 7.3).

Interaction	Skills
As a priority, you will need to understand the levels of risk; does his voice command him to act against himself or anyone else?	Harm reduction Personal safety
To achieve this, you would need to use a combination of interpersonal skills: • non-verbal cues (eye contact, non-threatening body position, facial expression and use of personal space); • verbal skills (calm and quiet tones, prompts, reflection, open questions, summarising or probing). Demonstrates a non-judgemental and genuine interest in Ed and his experiences. Being genuinely interested or curious in Ed's experiences can assist in developing a rapport enabling greater exploration of Ed's voices.	Interpersonal skills
Ed believes the alcohol and cannabis help create a sense of calm, suppressing negative thoughts and voices. By exploring with Ed his positive beliefs about cannabis and drug use you can establish his knowledge and his potential for change. Recognising that Ed may have a different understanding about how his dual diagnosis interacts than you do can help establish his knowledge, potential for psycho-educational approaches and his potential for change.	Person-centred approach Change theory Motivation for change Interpersonal skills Psycho-education
In developing the conversation, you might ask Ed about any negative experiences linked to his substance use. This will help you establish: • potential withdrawal problems from the alcohol; • a link between alcohol and voice hearing; • a link between cannabis and paranoia or voice hearing.	Motivational interviewing Change theory Physical care
You might re-examine this by exploring with Ed any changes in his voice (tone, language or volume) when he uses alcohol, or if his voice is different if he uses cannabis.	Motivational interviewing Psycho-education Interpersonal skills
Using your communication skills and curiosity can help you to ask and understand if Ed might be contemplating change. There may be the opportunity to decrease ambivalence in Ed's beliefs about his dual diagnosis.	Interpersonal skills Motivation for change

Table 7.2: Possible interventions for Ed

Interaction	Skills
If Ed is using alcohol on a daily basis, you would need to know: • the strength of the alcohol; • the amount he drinks per day; • when he has his first and last drink; • is this the same every day. This helps you to elicit the level of alcohol dependency and the potential withdrawal he will experience if he makes any changes.	The goal here is linked to safety, so you might consider using a psycho-educational (PE) or harm minimisation approach (HM)
If Ed is willing to change his alcohol use, based on your assessment of his level of dependency, you would help Ed prepare for any withdrawal symptoms. If he is likely to have withdrawal symptoms that need monitoring you could collaborate with a local alcohol service and support Ed to make contact.	Psycho-educational Interpersonal skills Change theory Signposting

Table 7.3: Revised plan for Ed

Activity 7.6   *Decision making*

There are many different patterns for substance use ranging from abstinent to dependency. What level of alcohol dependency is Ed?

Social use   Regular use   Heavy use   Dependent use

Based on your knowledge of Ed's alcohol use, if he suddenly stops drinking alcohol, what physical and psychological symptoms might he experience?

You will find some comments at the end of the chapter.

If Ed continues to use cannabis, what might you do? Taking a non-judgemental approach to what Ed is saying is critical; when this is combined with involving Ed in discussing safer cannabis use, reducing the harm potential, you are using an HR approach. You may be surprised to learn that increasing knowledge about the substance in every way is considered HR. Discussing with Ed how much he might smoke or buy, smoking in a safe environment or consuming cannabis to avoid smoking related harm and awareness of the legal implications for cannabis use are all HR and educational strategies. For mental health nurses you might have noticed that HR employs similar principles to working with voices (Intervoice, 2014).

Am I promoting continued substance use?

Harm reduction is not without controversy; it does not presume a goal of abstinence, taking a pragmatic approach that includes providing safe injecting spaces, clean needles or consumption rooms. This approach is aligned to health promotion and public health strategies (EMCDDA, 2010). Harm reduction does not encourage, promote or condone substance use or behaviours; rather it accepts this behaviour will occur and seeks to incrementally reduce adverse outcomes. In Ed's case an HR approach would accept that he does not want to make changes to his cannabis use, but is willing to make changes to his alcohol use. Taking this approach would enable support and information that promotes change over the longer term – small gains rather than immediate big changes.

You may find that Ed does not want any help and this can be difficult to accept. Ed might have some specific reasons for his decision: he may be concerned about being admitted to hospital or worried that stopping cannabis and alcohol will make his experience of voices worse. Be prepared to discuss these concerns with Ed; some of this may be based on mistaken assumptions. It can sometimes be easier to prepare and make changes when you are aware of what may happen. For Ed, this could mean understanding alcohol withdrawal might increase his feelings of depression, or make his voices louder, but that this is often temporary and begins to reduce within 72 hours. It may help Ed to know that there is medication he can use to help him through alcohol withdrawal; he might consider using family support, friendships or support groups like the Hearing Voices Network to help him develop new strategies for coping. You will need to have contact details for local services or be able to access these prior to, or as you discuss this with Ed.

Developing confidence and skills to work alone

No matter where you are in your professional development, a first year student or a registered nurse, you are constantly learning. Factual knowledge can be learned, new skills practised and developed over time building your competency and confidence – learning to work with dual diagnosis patients is no exception to this. As a nurse you are often the first contact point a patient might meet, and there are many skills that you have that can be used in assessing and interacting with dual diagnosis patients, but you would not be expected to work in isolation. The complex interactions that can occur in dual diagnosis require us to collaborate and share our expertise; we do not have to work in isolation, however we do have to improve our basic knowledge and skills.

The intensity of emotions we can experience demands we find ways to maintain our compassion and integrity, and collaborating with patients and colleagues is central to achieving this. The discomfort that we experience between our personal beliefs and professional roles coupled with a lack of immediate and visible results in working with dual diagnosis can lead to a culture of feeling de-skilled. Collaborating across disciplines enables supported practice;

prospects for clinical supervision with increased opportunities for learning from each other and the patients can in the longer term help improve cultural competence and therapeutic optimism (Rasool, 2006). As nurses we benefit and importantly so do the dual diagnosis patients we interact with.

Chapter summary

The emphasis in this chapter has been on exploring knowledge and skills nurses can use in interacting and working with dual diagnosis patients. Dual diagnosis is a highly prevalent global issue that continues to attract considerable stigma and debate from professionals and non-professionals alike. In every area of healthcare, you can expect to meet, provide nursing care or interact with a patient or relative who has a dual diagnosis. There is no typical dual diagnosis patient to guide our practice, and our tendency to focus on the most complex of cases (those patients requiring specialist mental health or addictions intervention) fuels our fears and frustrations, feeding our negative perceptions of the dual diagnosis patient group.

Developing dual diagnosis skills begins with our own education; increasing our knowledge of drugs, alcohol and mental health is a first step in building confidence and competence in working with multiple aspects of dual diagnosis nursing. You will nurse some dual diagnosis patients who are able to act on health promotion advice without assistance, while at the other end of the spectrum there are more complex patients whose mental health and substance use are so tangled and enmeshed that a collaborative team approach is needed. As a student nurse you will encounter many different dual diagnosis presentations along this spectrum. Being able to make sense of the links and associations between mental health and substance use builds confidence, and knowing how to access information, professional support or joint collaborative working is equally important.

Activities: brief outline answers

Activity 7.2 Reflection

You may have discovered that you hold some strong opinions or views about dual diagnosis patients. You may not have been aware that there are consistent reports of older adults using and misusing drugs and alcohol, which complicate physical and psychological health (Trevisan, 2014; NHS Choices, 2011). Social views of drugs and drug use are predominantly negative; most substance users are considered to be deceitful and make selfish lifestyle choices, with only themselves to blame. Health professionals are distrustful of the behaviours of people using drugs, often viewing them as manipulative and linked to choice (like recreational drug use), therefore the consequences become self-inflected (Lloyd, 2011). Substance use and mental health have associations in the public mind with danger and violence towards others; as a combination there is an assumption that this doubles the risk. While this may be true for some individuals, for the majority of people with either mental health or substance use problems this is more likely to reflect the stigma associated with either disorder.

Activity 7.3 Evidence-based practice and research

	Effects in intoxication	Effects in withdrawal
Stimulant drugs High energy drinks (Red Bull) or other caffeinated drinks Khat Cocaine and crack cocaine Amphetamine/meth-amphetamine	In the short term you might expect to see increased energy including an inability to remain still. You may observe body tension, restlessness or agitation. You would expect to see euphoria, however mood swings, anxiety and paranoia can also be present. You may find that speech is rapid, often jumping from topic to topic. Stimulant use can suppress hunger and thirst with associated weight loss, and poor sleep with insomnia is frequently observed. Stimulants act to increase blood pressure (hypertension) and pulse rate. You are likely to observe dilated pupils, and the experience of chest pain is not uncommon. Long-term use can lead to chest pain and cardiac complications including strokes occurring due to chronic hypertension and tachycardia. Arrhythmia and myocardial infarctions can occur.	Effects in withdrawal include: Slowed speech and sudden drops in energy (crash) with fatigue can occur – some individuals may sleep for considerable periods of time. Motor activity is reduced and the person's mood can become irritable and depressed. Suicidal thoughts and actions can occur, alongside paranoid thinking. Stimulant users can experience intense drug craving.
Depressant drugs Alcohol Diazepam (and other drugs belonging to the same drug family) Heroin (and other opiate-based drugs)	You are likely to observe a range of symptoms from drowsiness, mild sedation or unconsciousness or coma. Speech is slurred, and their subjective mood and energy is low, there are impairments to judgement (including sexual disinhibition) and reaction times can be slowed down. Irritable mood, confusion and memory loss can be present. Physically, people can experience nausea and vomiting, lowering of blood pressure, pulse and body temperature. In cases of overdose, respiration rates are suppressed, cyanosis is present. Longer term effects are often drug dependent, however depressant drugs have been associated with liver disease (alcohol), depression, respiratory and pancreatic problems and death including accidental overdose.	Withdrawal symptoms can range from mild to severe, linked to the drug choice and dose. Psychologically, you might expect to see anxiety, irritability, agitation or paranoia in the initial phase. Panic attacks are not uncommon. Physically symptoms of nausea or vomiting, sweats, muscle twitches or spasm, insomnia are frequently seen, and some people can experience withdrawal seizures. Severe alcohol withdrawal can be fatal.

	Effects in intoxication	Effects in withdrawal
Psychedelic drugs LSD Ecstasy Ketamine Magic mushrooms	Symptoms of intoxication range from mild alteration of perceptions (sight, sound, feeling and touch), time distortion and feeling spiritually aware to negative experiences of hallucinations, or extreme anxiety, paranoia or delusions. You would expect to see pupil dilation, hypertension, accelerated pulse and a lowering of body temperature. Some people may experience jaw clenching, excess salivation and sweating. Insomnia and tremors can also be associated with some psychedelic drugs. Psychedelic drug users may come to services due to accidental injuries as a result of their intoxication.	Psychedelics are generally considered non-addictive, there is a gradual reduction of intoxication effects, and the body functions usually return to normal (homeostasis). Occasionally some users can experience psychotic symptoms beyond the drug withdrawal phase.
Other Solvent	Intoxication symptoms are similar to alcohol with many solvents acting as central nervous system depressants. Psychological effects include initial feelings of euphoria and decreased inhibitions; however, disorientation, agitation and aggression do occur. Hallucinations can occur, however these are drug dependent. Physically, you would expect to see uncoordinated gait, nose bleeds, nausea and vomiting. There can be skin irritation around the mouth or nose. Solvent users can be at increased risk of death due to sudden blockage of airways, heart failure or asphyxiation of vomit. Long-term use can cause recurrent chest infections, weight loss, blackouts and seizures.	Withdrawal symptoms can vary from person to person and are linked to the type of solvent used. You might expect to see anxiety attacks, muscle tension, depression and insomnia. Headaches, dry cough, nausea, and vomiting with weight loss are some of the physical effects experienced; however, some solvents can cause chest pain and dizziness. Insomnia is likely to occur along with intense drug cravings.

Activity 7.5 Critical thinking

Ed has a previous diagnosis of schizophrenia; his current mental health issues include: altered perceptions, auditory hallucinations and paranoia, he is isolating himself from family and social networks and is experiencing suicidal thinking which could be related to either his voice hearing or a possible depression. Ed is currently using alcohol and cannabis on a daily basis. As his mental health triggers his use of alcohol and cannabis, and the alcohol and cannabis are increasing his mental health symptomatology, Ed would meet criteria for a complex dual diagnosis.

Activity 7.6 Decision making

You have been made aware that Ed uses alcohol and cannabis daily.

You may have discovered the sensible drinking limits for men is three to four units per day (Ed is drinking more than this – four cans of 8 per cent lager per day, estimated at 20 units of alcohol/day, and 140 units/week), so it is likely Ed will have developed a physical and psychological tolerance, and highly likely that Ed would experience physical and psychological withdrawals if he suddenly stops drinking (Drinkaware, 2014). If Ed is unaware of these possible effects, he may link withdrawal symptoms to his mental health, reinforcing any negative views he has about his mental health.

If Ed were to suddenly stop his alcohol use, it is likely that he would experience alcohol withdrawal symptoms, including tremors, shaking, sweating, nausea, possible vomiting or withdrawal seizures. He is likely to become hypersensitive to noise and light with headaches. Ed would experience poor sleep and appetite during the first week which could enhance his mental health issues including his experience of voices, paranoia, anxiety and depression. As he experiences altered perceptions (auditory voice) he is at increased risk of additional hallucinations (particularly auditory, visual or tactile). Psychologically, any symptoms of anxiety experienced by Ed would be magnified during the first 72 hours; he is likely to be irritable and agitated (which may not necessarily be related to his mental health). Ed might find that his experience of voices is more persistent, louder, last longer and more negative in tone.

Further reading

Denning, P, Little, J and Glickman, A (2005) *Over the Influence: The harm reduction guide for managing drugs and alcohol.* New York: Guilford Press.

An introductory guide to the principles and practice of harm reduction, promoting a patient-centred and compassionate approach to working with addictions, and how we might encourage people to change.

Department of Health (2002) *Mental Health Policy Implementation Guide: Dual diagnosis good practice guidance.* London: DH.

This guidance remains the principal document for defining dual diagnosis; summarising good practice in assessment and treatment in the United Kingdom context.

Miller, R and Rollnick, S (2012) *Motivational Interviewing: Helping People Change (Applications of Motivational Interviewing),* 3rd edition. New York: Guilford Press.

An introductory text on developing and using motivational interviewing skills in practice; it is one of the key approaches in working with dual diagnosis and substance use patients.

Pycroft, A (2012) *Understanding and Working with Substance Misusers.* London: Sage.

This is an informative and easy read for anyone interested in working with addictions. The main philosophies and treatment in addictions are explored, helping to develop basic addictions knowledge which will support and enhance your interventions with dual diagnosis patients.

Rassool, HG (2009) *Dual Diagnosis Nursing.* Oxford: Blackwell Publishing.

This book provides clinicians with contemporary treatment approaches from theoretical and clinical perspectives specific to dual diagnosis within a UK perspective.

Useful websites

www.dualdiagnosis.co.uk

The National Consortium for Dual Diagnosis Nurse Consultants: The website provides information from clinicians working in dual diagnosis; resources available include information for professionals, carers and patients.

www.erowid.org

Erowid: This database manages a vast source of drug and alcohol information, including a dictionary of different drugs, how they work and drug user perspectives.

www.nice.org.uk

National Institute of Clinical Excellence (NICE): This site provides guidance and standards for drugs, alcohol, mental health and dual diagnosis practice and treatment within the UK.

www.turning-point.co.uk

Turning Point is one of the largest charitable service providers in addiction and dual diagnosis treatment in the UK. The website hosts a rich source of information, blogs and toolkits.

References

Abba, N, Chadwick, P and Stevenson, C (2008) Responding mindfully to distressing psychosis: A grounded theory analysis. *Psychotherapy Research*, 18(1): 77–87.

Amer, M (2006) Cannabinoids in medicine: A review of their therapeutic potential. *Journal of Ethnopharmacology*, 105: 1–25.

American Psychiatric Association (APA) (2000) *Diagnostic and Statistical Manual of Mental Disorders, Fourth Edition: DSM-IV-TR®*. Arlington, VA: American Psychiatric Association.

Anderson, C, Hogarty, G and Reiss, D (1981) The psychoeducational family treatment of schizophrenia. *New Directions for Mental Health Services*, 12: 79–94.

Anxiety Care UK (2014) *The Biological Effects and Consequences of Anxiety*. Available online at: http://www.anxietycare.org.uk/docs/biologicaleffects.asp (accessed March 2014).

Appleby, L (2007) *Mental Health Ten Years On: Progress on mental health care reform*. Available online at: http://webarchive.nationalarchives.gov.uk/20130107105354/http://www.dh.gov.uk/prod_consum_dh/groups/dh_digitalassets/@dh/@en/documents/digitalasset/dh_074235.pdf (accessed March 2014).

Arria, A and DuPont, R (2010) Nonmedical prescription stimulant use among college students: Why we need to do something and what we need to do. *Journal of Addiction Studies*, 29(4): 417–26.

Bach, S and Grant, A (2009) *Communication and Interpersonal Skills in Nursing*, 2nd edition. Exeter: Learning Matters.

Baker, D, Pryce, G, Giovannoni, G and Thompson, A (2003) The therapeutic potential of cannabis. *The Lancet*, 2: 291.

Bandelow, B, Schmahl, C, Falkai, P and Wedekind, D (2010) Borderline personality disorder: A dysregulation of the endogenous opioid system? *Psychological Review*, 117(2): 623–36.

Bartsch, A, Homola, G, Biller, A, Smith, S, Weijers, G, Wiesbeck, G, Jenkinson, M, De Stefano, N, Solymosil, L and Bendszus, M (2007) Manifestations of early brain recovery associated with abstinence from alcohol. *Brain*, 130: 36–47.

Beck, AT (1963) Thinking and depression: I. Idiosyncratic content and cognitive distortions. *Archives of General Psychiatry*, 9: 324–33.

Beck, A (1976) *Cognitive Therapy and the Emotional Disorders*. New York: International Universities Press.

Bell, AC and D'Zurilla, TJ (2009) Problem-solving therapy for depression: A meta-analysis. *Clinical Psychology Review*, 29: 348–53.

Bennett-Levy, J, Turner, F, Beaty, T, Smith, M, Paterson, B and Farmer, S (2001) The value of self-practice of cognitive therapy techniques and self-reflection in the training of cognitive therapists. *Behavioural and Cognitive Psychotherapy*, 29: 203–20.

Bennett-Levy, J, Richards, DA and Farrand, P (2010) Low intensity CBT interventions: A revolution in mental health care, in Bennett-Levy et al. (eds) *Oxford Guide to Low Intensity CBT Interventions*. Oxford: Oxford University Press.

Blair, SN and Morris, JN (2009) Healthy hearts – and the universal benefits of being physically active: Physical activity and health. *Annals of Epidemiology*, 19(4): 253–56.

British Liver Trust (2014) *Alcohol*. Available online at: http://www.britishlivertrust.org.uk/liver-information/liver-conditions/alcohol (accessed 23 May 2011).

British Medical Association (BMA) (2013) *Drugs of Dependence: The role of medical professionals*. London: BMA Board of Science.

Brousselle, A, Lamothe, L, Mercier, C and Perreault, M (2007) Beyond limitations of best practice: How logic analysis helped reinterpret dual diagnosis guidelines. *Evaluation and Programme Planning*, 30: 94–104.

Business Wire (2014) *Alkermes announces initiation of ALKS 5461 pivotal clinical program for Treatment of Major Depressive Disorder*. Available online at: http://www.businesswire.com/news/home/20140306005375/en/.U4SpZPnGr4I (accessed 27 May 2014).

Butler, AC and Beck, AT (1995) Cognitive therapy for depression. *The Clinical Psychologist*, 48: 3–5.

Cannaway, R and Merkes, M (2010) Barriers to comorbidity service delivery: The complexities of dual diagnosis and the need to agree on terminology and conceptual frameworks. *Australian Health Review*, 34: 262–8.

Chadwick, P (2006) *Person-Based Cognitive Therapy for Distressing Voices*. Chichester: Wiley.

Cohen, M, Solowij, N and Carr, V (2008) Cannabis, cannabinoids and schizophrenia: Integration of the evidence. *Australian and New Zealand Journal of Psychiatry*, 42: 357–68.

Coombes, L and Wratten, A (2007) The lived experience of community mental health nurses working with people who have dual diagnosis: A phenomenological study. *Journal of Psychiatric and Mental Health Nursing*, 14: 382–92.

Cuijpers, P, van Straten, A and Warmerdam, L (2007a) Behavioral activation treatments of depression: A meta-analysis. *Clinical Psychology Review*, 27: 318–26.

Cuijpers, P, van Straten, A and Warmerdam, L (2007b) Problem solving therapies for depression: A meta-analysis. *European Psychiatry*, 22: 9–15.

Deans, C and Soar, R (2005) Caring for clients with dual diagnosis in rural communities in Australia: The experience of mental health professionals. *Journal of Psychiatric and Mental Health Nursing*, 12: 268–74.

Department of Health (DH) (2002) *Mental Health Policy Implementation Guide: Dual diagnosis good practice guide*. London: DH.

Department of Health (DH) (2011a) *Talking Therapies: A four year plan of action*. London: DH.

Department of Health (DH) (2011b) *Start Active, Stay Active: A report on physical activity from the four home countries' Chief Medical Officers.* London: Stationery Office.

Dimeff, L and Linehan, M (2001) Dialectical behavior therapy in a nutshell. *The Californian Psychologist,* 34: 10–13.

Disability Rights Commission (DRC) (2006) *Equal Treatment: Closing the gap – information for people with learning disabilities and/or mental health problems and other disabled people.* London: Disability Rights Commission.

Drinkaware (2013) *Alcohol and Mental Health Factsheet.* Available online at: http://www.drinkaware. co.uk/check-the-facts/health-effects-of-alcohol/mental-health/alcohol-and-mental-health (accessed 24 May 2014).

Drinkaware (2014) *Check the Facts/Health Effects of Alcohol.* Available online at: https://www. drinkaware.co.uk (accessed 2 June 2014).

Dunkley, C (2012) http://www.sfdbt.com (accessed 13 March 2013).

Edward, K and Munro, I (2009) Nursing considerations for dual diagnosis in mental health. *Journal of Nursing Practice,* 15: 74–9.

Edward, K and Robin, A (2012) Dual diagnosis, as described by those who experience the disorder: Using the Internet as a source of data. *International Journal of Mental Health Nursing,* 21: 550–9.

European Monitoring Centre for Drugs and Drug Addiction (EMCDDA) (2010) *Harm Reduction: Evidence, impacts and challenges. Monograph 10.* Available online at. file:///C:/Users/kim/Downloads/EMCDDA-monograph10-harm%20reduction_final.pdf (accessed 2 June 2014).

European Monitoring Centre for Drugs and Drug Addiction (EMCDDA) (2011) *Synthetic Cannabinoids and Spice.* Available online at: http://www.emcdda.europa.eu/publications/drug-profiles/synthetic-cannabinoids (accessed 8 June 2014).

European Monitoring Centre for Drugs and Drug Addiction (EMCDDA) (2012) *2012 Annual Report on the State of the Drugs Problem in Europe.* Available online at: http://www.emcdda.europa. eu/publications/annual-report/2012 (accessed 2 September 2014).

Farb, NAS, Anderson, AK, Mayberg, H, Bean, J, McKeon, D and Segal, ZV (2010) Minding one's emotions: Mindfulness training alters the neural expression of sadness. *Emotion,* 10(1): 25–33.

Feigenbaum, JD, Fonagy, P, Pilling, S, Jones, A, Wildgoose, A and Bebbington, PE (2012) A real-world study of the effectiveness of DBT in the UK National Health Service. *British Journal of Clinical Psychology,* 51: 121–41.

Finn, D and Crabbe, J (1997) Exploring alcohol withdrawal syndrome. *Alcohol, Health and Research World,* 21(2): 149–56.

Glaucoma Research Foundation (2013) *Should You Be Smoking Marijuana to Treat Your Glaucoma?* Available online at: http://www.glaucoma.org/treatment/should-you-be-smoking-marijuana-to-treat-your-glaucoma-1.php (accessed 18 June 2014).

Godfrin, K and van Heeringen, C (2010) The effects of mindfulness-based cognitive therapy on recurrence of depressive episodes, mental health and quality of life: A randomised controlled study. *Behaviour Research and Therapy,* 48(8): 738–46.

Grossman, P (2004) Mindfulness-based stress reduction and health benefits: A meta-analysis. *Journal of Psychosomatic Research*, 57(1): 35–43.

Gumley, A, Taylor, H, Schwannauer, M and MacBeth, A (2013) A systematic review of attachment and psychosis: Measurement, construct validity and outcomes. *Acta Psychiatrica Scandinavica*, 129(4): 257–74.

Harker, R (2012) *Statistics on Alcohol 2009/10. Standard Note: SN/SG/3311.* London: House of Commons Library.

Hawn, G (2011) *10 Mindful Minutes.* London: Routledge.

Hayes, S and Stroshal, K (eds) (2004) *A Practical Guide to Acceptance and Commitment Therapy.* New York: Guilford Press.

Hoffman, PD, Fruzetti, AE and Swenson, CR (1999) Dialectical behavior therapy: Family skills training. *Family Process*, 38(4): 399.

Hopko, DR, Lejuez, CW, Ruggiero, KJ and Eifert, GH (2003) Contemporary behavioral activation treatments for depression: Procedures, principles, and progress. *Clinical Psychology Review*, 23: 699–717.

Huntley, Z, Maltezos, S, Williams, C, Morinan, A, Hammon, A, Ball, D, Marshall, E, Keaney, F, Young, S, Bolton, P, Glaser, K, Howe-Forbes, R, Kuntsi, J, Xenitidis, K, Murphy, D and Asherson, P (2012) Rates of undiagnosed attention deficit hyperactivity disorder in London drug and alcohol detoxification units. *Biomed Central, Psychiatry*. Available online at: http://www.biomedcentral.com/content/pdf/1471–244X-12–223.pdf (accessed 27 May 2014).

Ingram, RE and Luxton, D (2005) Vulnerability-stress models, in Hankin, BE and Abela, J (eds) *Development of Psychopathology: A vulnerability-stress perspective*, Chapter 2. London: Sage.

Ingram, R and Price, J (eds) (2010) *Vulnerability to Psychopathology: Risk across the lifespan.* London: Sage.

Ingram, R, Atchley, R and Segal, Z (2011) *Vulnerability to Depression: From cognitive neuroscience to prevention and treatment.* New York: Guilford Press.

Intervoice (2014) A practical guide to coping with voices. *The International Hearing Voices Network*. Available online at: http://www.intervoiceonline.org/support-recovery/a-practical-guide (accessed 2 June 2014).

Kabat-Zinn, J (2003) Mindfulness-based interventions in context: Past, present and future. *Clinical Psychology: Science and Practice*, 10(2): 144–56.

Katzmarzyk, PT (2010) Physical activity, sedentary behavior, and health: Paradigm paralysis or paradigm shift? *Diabetes*, 59(11): 2717–25.

Kensinger, E (2007) Negative emotion enhances memory accuracy: Behavioral and neuroimaging evidence. *Current Directions in Psychological Science*, 16(4): 213–8.

King's Fund (2008) *Paying the Price: The cost of mental health care in England to 2026.* London: King's Fund.

Kitchner, B, Jorm, A and Lubman, D (2011) Mental health: Substance use first aid, in Cooper, D (ed) *Responding in Mental Health and Substance Use.* London: Radcliffe Publishing, pp 101–18.

Kristeller, JL and Hallett, CB (1999) An exploratory study of a meditation-based intervention for binge eating disorder. *Journal of Health Psychology*, 4(3): 357–63.

Kweskin, S (2013) The dope on medical cannabis: Results of a survey of psychiatrists. *Psychiatric Times*. Available online at: http://www.psychiatrictimes.com (accessed 26 May 2014).

Lanktree, C and Briere, J (2008) *Integrative Treatment of Complex Trauma for Children Ages 8 to 12 (ITCT-C)*. Long Beach, CA: MCAVIC-USC Child and Adolescent Trauma Program, National Child Traumatic Stress Network, Substance Abuse and Mental Health Services Administration, U.S. Department of Health and Human Services.

Linehan, M (1993a) *Skills Training Manual for Treating Borderline Personality Disorder: Diagnosis and treatment of mental disorders (diagnosis and treatment of mental disorders)*. New York: Guilford Press.

Linehan, M (1993b) *Cognitive-Behavioral Treatment of Boderline Personality Disorder*. New York: Guildford Press.

Linehan, MM (2003a) *Skills Training Manual for Treating Borderline Personality Disorder*. New York: Guilford Press.

Linehan, MM (2003b) *Cognitive Behavioral Treatment of Borderline Personality Disorder*. New York: Guilford Press.

Linehan, M, Armstrong, HE, Suarez, A, Allmon, D and Heard, HL (1991) Cognitive-behavioral treatment of chronically parasuicidal borderline patients. *Archives of General Psychiatry*, 48: 1060–4.

Little, SE (2009) The Therapeutic Relationship in Dialectical Behavior Therapy: A Longitudinal Investigation in a Naturalistic Setting *Dissertations (2009–)*. Paper 160. http://epublications.marquette.edu/dissertations_mu/160 (accessed 13 March 2013).

Lloyd, C (2011) *Sinning and Sinned Against: The stigmatisation of problem drug users*. London: United Kingdom Drug Policy Commission.

Locke, EAS, Karyll, N, Saari, Lise, M and Latham, GP (1981) Goal setting and task performance. *Psychological Bulletin*, 90: 125–52.

Lovi, R and Barr, J (2009) Stigma reported by nurses related to those experiencing drug and alcohol dependency: A phenomenological Giorgi study. *Contemporary Nurse*, 33(2): 166–78.

Lynch, T and Robins, C (1997) Treatment of borderline personality disorder using dialectical behavior therapy. *Journal of the California Alliance for the Mentally Ill*, 8(1): 47–9.

McCabe, M, Straiger, P, Thomas, A, Cross, W and Ricciardelli, L (2011) Screening for comorbid substance use disorders among people with mental health diagnosis who present to emergency departments. *Australasian Emergency Nursing Journal*, 14: 163–71.

McKay, M, Wood, JC and Brantley, J (2007) *The Dialectical Behavior Therapy Skills Workbook*. Oakland, CA: New Harbinger.

Mancebo, M, Grant, J, Pinto, A, Eisen, J and Rassmussen, S (2009) Substance use disorders in obsessive compulsive disorder clinical sample. *Journal of Anxiety Disorders*, 23: 429–35.

Meaux, J, Hester, C, Smith, B and Shoptaw, A (2006) Stimulant medications: A trade off? The lived experience of adolescents with ADHD. *Journal of Specialists in Paediatric Nursing*, 11(4): 214–26.

Mental Health Policy Group, London School of Economics (LSE) (2012) *How Mental Illness Loses Out in the NHS*. London: LSE.

Miller, B and Rollnick, S (2012) *Meeting in the Middle: Motivational interviewing and self determination theory*. Available online at: http://www.ijbnpa.org/content/pdf/1479–5868–9–25.pdf (accessed 31 May 2014).

Moore, K and Rassool, HG (2008) Addiction and mental health nursing: A synthesis of role and care in the community, in Rassool, HG (ed) *Dual Diagnosis Nursing*. Oxford: Blackwell Science Publication.

Morris, JN and Crawford, MD (1958) Coronary heart disease and physical activity of work. *British Medical Journal*, 2(5111): 1485–96.

Muller-Vahl, K, Theloe, K, Kolbe, K, Emrich, H and Schineider, U (2003) Treatment of Tourette Syndrome with Delta-9-Tetrahydrocannabinol (D9-THC): No influence on neuropsychological performance. *Neuropsychopharmacology*, 28: 384–8.

Mynors-Wallis, LM, Gath, D, Day, A and Baker, F (2000) Randomised controlled trial of problem-solving treatment, antidepressant medication and combined treatment for major depression in primary care. *British Medical Journal*, 320: 26–30.

Nash, JM (1997) Addicted. *Time*, 149(18): 69–76.

New, A and Stanley, B (2010) An opioid deficit in borderline personality disorder: Self-cutting, substance use and social dysfunction. *American Journal of Psychiatry*, 167: 882–5.

New Zealand Asthma Foundation (2010) *Cannabis and the Lung*. Available online at: http://asthmafoundation.org.nz/wp-content/uploads/2012/03/Cannabis.pdf (accessed 26 May 2014).

NHS Choices (2011) *Elderly 'Need Drug and Alcohol Support'*. Available online at: http://www.nhs.uk/news/2011/06June/Pages/drink-limits-for-over-65s.aspx (accessed 23 May 2014).

NHS Choices (2014) *Could a Compound in Cannabis Treat Epilepsy?* Available online at: http://www.nhs.uk/news/2014/05May/Pages/Could-a-compound-found-in-cannabis-treat-epilepsy.aspx (accessed 23 May 2014).

National Collaborating Centre for Mental Health (NCCMH) (2010) *Depression: The NICE guideline on the treatment and management of depression in adults*. Updated edition. London: BPS and RCPSYCH.

National Collaborating Centre for Mental Health (NCCMH) (2014) *Psychosis and Schizophrenia in Adults: Treatment and management*. London: National Institute for Health and Care Excellence.

National Institute for Health and Care Excellence (NICE) (2009) *Treatment Guidelines for Borderline Personality Disorder*. London: NICE.

National Institute for Health and Care Excellence (NICE) (2011) *Commissioning Stepped Care for People with Common Mental Health Disorders*. London: DH. Available online at: http://publications.nice.org.uk/commissioning-stepped-care-for-people-with-common-mental-health-disorders-cmg41/3-a-stepped-care-approach-to-commissioning-high-quality-integrated-care-for-people-with-common (accessed March 2014).

National Institute for Health and Care Excellence (NICE) (2014) *Alcohol-Use Disorders Pathway*. National Institute for Health Care and Excellence. Available online at: http://pathways.nice.org.uk/pathways/alcohol-use-disorders (accessed 24 May 2014).

National Institute for Health and Care Excellence (NICE, N.I.F.H.A.C.E.) (2009) Depression. The NICE guideline on the treatment and management of depression in adults, in HEALTH, N. C. C. F. M. (ed). Great Britain: Stanley Hunt.

National Institute for Health and Care Excellence (NICE, N.I.F.H.A.C.E.) (2011) Generalised anxiety disorder and panic disorder (with or without agoraphobia) in adults (CG113).

Ng, B and O'Brien, A (2009) Beyond ADHD and narcolepsy: Psychostimulants in general psychiatry. *Advances in Psychiatric Treatment,* 15: 297–305.

Nuechterlein, K and Dawson, ME (1984) A heuristic vulnerability/stress model of schizophrenic episodes. *Schizophrenia Bulletin,* 10(2): 300–12.

Nursing and Midwifery Council (NMC) (2002) *The Recognition, Prevention and Therapeutic Management of Violence in Mental Health Care. A Summary.* UK: United Kingdom Central Council for Nursing, Midwifery and Health Visiting.

Nursing and Midwifery Council (NMC) (2008) *The Code: Standards of conduct, performance and ethics for nurses and midwives.* Available online at: http://www.nmc-uk.org/Publications/Standards/The-code/Introduction

O'Donovan et al. (2010) The ABC of physical activity for health: A consensus statement from the British Association of Sport and Exercise Sciences. *Journal of Sport Sciences,* 28(6): 573–91.

Ohlmeier, M, Peters, K, Wild, B, Zedler, M and Ziegenbein, M (2008) Comorbidity of alcohol and substance dependence with attention-deficit/hyperactivity disorder (ADHD). *Alcohol and Alcoholism,* 43(3): 300–4.

Orozco, LJ, Buchleitner, AM, Gimenez-Perez, G, Roque i Figuls, M, Richter, B and Mauricio, D (2008) Exercise or exercise and diet for preventing type 2 diabetes mellitus (Review). *The Cochrane Collaboration.*

Padesky, CA and Greenberger, D (1996) *Mind over Mood.* New York: Guilford Press.

Palmer, RL, Birchall, H, Damani, S, Gatward, N, McGrain, L and Parker, L (2003) A dialectical behavior therapy program for people with an eating disorder and borderline personality disorder: Description and outcome. *International Journal of Eating Disorders,* 33(3): 281–6.

Papworth, M, Marrinan, T, Martin, B, Keegan, D and Chaddock, A (2013) *Low Intensity Cognitive Behaviour Therapy: A Practitioners Guide.* London: Sage.

Parakh, P and Basu, D (2013) Cannabis and psychosis: Have we found the missing links? *Asian Journal of Psychiatry,* 6: 281–7.

Phillips, P (2007) Dual diagnosis: An exploratory qualitative study of staff perceptions of substance misuse among the mentally ill in Northern India. *Issues in Mental Health Nursing,* 28: 1309–22.

Prochaska, J and DiClimente, C (1982) Transtheoretical therapy: Toward a more integrative model of change. *Psychotherapy Theory, Research and Practice,* 19(3): 276–88.

Quantum, T (2014) *Mindfulness Meditation for PTSD, TBI and Compassion Fatigue.* New York: LLC.

Rani, S and Byrne, H (2012) A multi-method evaluation of a training course on dual diagnosis. *Journal of Psychiatric and Mental Health Nursing,* 19: 509–20.

Rassool, GH (ed) (2006) Understanding dual diagnosis: An overview, in *Dual Diagnosis Nursing*. Oxford: Blackwell Publishing.

Rassool, GH and Rawaf, S (2008) Predictors or educational outcomes of undergraduate nursing students in alcohol and drug education. *Nurse Education Today*, 28: 691–701.

Rassool, GH, Villar-Luis, M, Carraro, TE and Lopes, G (2006) Undergraduate nursing students' perceptions of substance use and misuse: A Brazilian position. *Journal of Psychiatric and Mental Health Nursing*, 13: 85–9.

Reddy, M, Anderson, B, Liebschutz, J and Stein, M (2013) Factor structure of PTSD symptoms in opioid-dependent patients rating their overall trauma history. *Drug and Alcohol Dependence*, 132: 597–602.

Rezek, CA (2012) *Brilliant Mindfulness*. Edinburgh: Pearson.

Richards, D and Whyte, M (2011) *Reach Out: National Programme Student Materials to Support the Delivery of Training for Psychological Wellbeing Practitioners Delivering Low Intensity Interventions*. London: Rethink.

Rogers, C (1995) *Client-Centered Therapy: Its current practice, implications, and theory*. London: Constable.

Rojas-Corrales, M, Gilbert-Rahola, J and Mico, J (2007) Role of atypical opiates in OCD: Experimental approach through the study of 5-HT2A/C receptor-mediated behavior. *Psychopharmacology*, 190: 221–31.

Royal College of Psychiatrists (RCP) (2013) *Alcohol and Depression*. Available online at: http://www.rcpsych.ac.uk/healthadvice/problemsdisorders/alcoholdepression.aspx (accessed 23 May 2014).

Royal College of Psychiatrists (RCP) (2014) *Alcohol: Our favourite drug*. Available online at: http://www.rcpsych.ac.uk/healthadvice/problemsdisorders/alcoholourfavouritedrug.aspx (accessed 12 May 2014).

Sadler, C (2006) Snowed under. *Nursing Standard*, 20(35): 22–4.

Sara, G, Burgess, P, Malhi, G, Whiteford, H and Hall, W (2013) Differences in associations between cannabis and stimulant disorders in first admission psychosis. *Schizophrenia Research*, 147: 216–22.

Segal, Z, Teasdale, J and Williams, M (2002) *Mindfulness-Based Cognitive Therapy for Depression*. New York: Guilford Press.

South Australia Health (SA Health) (2012) *A Framework for the Recognition and Management of Challenging Behaviour*. Adelaide: SA Health. Available online at: http://www.sahealth.sa.gov.au/wps/wcm/connect/8966f000414a7549a7c4af6e3bdc556a/2_RMCB_Framework_PHCS_SQ_20130930.pdf?MOD=AJPERES&CACHEID=8966f000414a7549a7c4af6e3bdc556a (accessed January 2014).

Speca, M, Carlson, LE, Goodey, E and Angun, M (2000) A randomised, wait-list controlled clinical trial: The effect of a mindfulness meditation-based stress reduction program on mood and symptoms of stress in cancer outpatients. *Psychosomatic Medicine*, 62: 613–22.

Stefanis, N, Delespaul, P, Henquet, C, Bakoula, C, Stefanis, C and Van, J (2004) Early adolescent cannabis exposure and positive and negative dimensions of psychosis. *Society for the Study of Addiction*, 99: 1333–41.

Stotz, G, Woggon, B and Angst, J (1999) Psychostimulants in the therapy of treatment resistant depression: Review of the literature and findings from a retrospective study in 65 depressed patients. *Clinical Neuorscience*, 1(3): 165–74.

Swales, MA and Heard, HL (2007). The therapy relationship in dialectical behaviour therapy, in Gilbert, P and Leahy, R (eds) *The Therapeutic Relationship in the Cognitive Behavioral Psychotherapies*. New York: Routledge.

Talimbekova, V and Nurkodiaev, S (2010) Personality disorders at opioid dependent. *Medical and Health Science Journal*, 2: 100–3.

Teasdale, JD, Segal, ZV, Williams, JMG, Ridgeway, VA, Soulsby, JM and Lau, MA (2000) Prevention of relapse/recurrence in major depression by mindfulness-based cognitive therapy. *Journal of Consulting and Clinical Psychology*, 68: 615–23.

Tolliver, B (2010) Bipolar disorder and substance abuse: Overcoming the challenges of dual diagnosis patients. *Current Psychiatry*, 9(8): 31–41.

Tomlinson, K, Tate, S, Anderson, K, McCarthy, D and Brown, S (2006) An examination of self-medication and rebound effects: Psychiatric symptomatology before and after alcohol and drug relapse. *Addictive Behaviour*, 31(3): 461–74.

Tran, D, Stone, A, Fernandez, R, Griffiths, R and Johnson, M (2009) Changes in general nurses' knowledge of alcohol and substance use and misuse after education. *Perspectives in Psychiatric Care*, 45(2): 128–39.

Trevisan, L (2014) Elderly alcohol use disorders: Epidemiology, screening and assessment issues. *Psychiatric Times*. Available online at: http://www.psychiatrictimes.com/alcohol-abuse/elderly-alcohol-use-disorders-epidemiology-screening-and-assessment-issues (accessed 20 June 2014).

United Kingdom Drug Policy Commission (UKDPC) (2012) *Dual Diagnosis: A challenge for the reformed NHS and for Public Health England: A discussion paper from Centre for Mental Health, DrugScope and UK Drug Policy Commission*. London: UKDPC.

United Kingdom Government (1971) *Misuse of Drugs Act*. United Kingdom Government Legislation.

United Kingdom Government (2000) *Parliamentary Memorandum. Select Committee on Health: Appendices to the minutes of evidence*. Available online at: http://www.publications.parliament.uk/pa/cm199900/cmselect/cmhealth/373/373ap21.htm (accessed 24 June 2014).

Von Korff, M and Tiemens, B (2000) Individualized stepped care of chronic illness. *Western Journal of Medicine*, 172(2): 133–7.

Waddell, K and Skärsäter, I (2007) Nurses' experience of caring for patients with a dual diagnosis of depression and alcohol abuse in a general psychiatric setting. *Issues in Mental Health Nursing*, 28: 1125–40.

Warburton, DER, Nicol, CW and Bredin, SSD (2006) Health benefits of physical activity: The evidence. *Canadian Medical Association Journal*, 174(6): 801–9.

Ware, M, Tongtong, W, Shapiro, S, Robinson, A, Ducruet, T, Huynh, T, Gamsa, A, Bennett, G and Collet, J-P (2010) Smoked cannabis for chronic neuropathic pain: A randomized controlled trial. *CMAJ*, 182(14): E694–E701.

Westbrook, D, Kennerly, H and Kirk, J (2011) *An Introduction to Cognitive Behaviour Therapy Skills and Applications*, 2nd edition. London: Sage.

Williams, C (2003) *Overcoming Anxiety: A five areas approach*. London: Arnold.

Williams, C (2009) *Overcoming Depression and Low Mood*, 3rd edition. London: Hodder Arnold.

Williams, C and Garland, A (2002) A cognitive-behavioural therapy assessment model for use in everyday clinical practice. *Advances in Psychiatric Treatment*, 8: 172–9.

Williams, M and Penman, D (2011) *Mindfulness: A practical guide to finding peace in a frantic world*. Great Britain: Piatkus.

Winder, G, Stern, N and Hosanger, A (2013) Are 'bathsalts' the next generation of stimulant abuse? *Journal of Substance Abuse Treatment*, 44: 42–5.

Wiplfi, BM, Rethorst, CD and Landers, D (2008) The anxiolytic effects of exercise: A meta-analysis of randomized trials and dose-response analysis. *Journal of Sport and Exercise Psychology*, 30(4): 392–410.

Witek-Janusek, A, Albuquerque, K, Chroniak, KR, Chroniak, C, Durazo, R and Matthews, HL (2008) Effect of mindfulness based stress reduction on immune function, quality of life and coping in women newly diagnosed with early stage breast cancer. *Brain, Behavior, and Immunity*, 22(6): 969–81.

Wolff, E, Gaudlitz, K, von Lindenberger, B-L, Plag, J, Heinz, A and Strohle, A (2011) Exercise and physical activity in mental disorders. *European Archive of Psychiatry and Clinical Neuroscience*, 261(Suppl. 2): 186–91.

World Health Organisation (WHO) (1992) *International Classification of Diseases*. Available online at: http://www.who.int/classifications/icd/en (accessed 12 May 2014).

World Health Organisation (WHO) (2010) *Global Recommendations on Physical Activity for Health*. Switzerland: WHO.

World Health Organisation (WHO) (2014) *Management of substance abuse: Lexicon of alcohol and drug terms published by the World Health Organisation*. Available online at: http://www.sho.int/substance_abuse/terminology/who_lexicon/en (accessed 24 May 2014).

Zgierska, A (2010) Mindfulness based therapies for substance use disorders. *Substance Abuse*, 31(2): 77–8.

Zubin, J and Spring, B (1977) Vulnerability: A new view on schizophrenia. *Journal of Abnormal Psychology*, 86: 103–26.

Index

A

acceptance and commitment therapy (ACT) 16, 17
'ACCEPTS' technique 44
acting opposite 52, 61
action plan 100
action urges 50–1, 52, 61
adaptive thoughts 120
addictions *see* dual diagnosis; substance abuse
Adler, A. 24
adrenaline 93
agenda setting 33
alcohol 103, 131–2, 133, 137, 143
   level of dependency 145
   withdrawal effects 132, 145
amphetamine 133, 143
anorexia nervosa 112
anxiety 83, 84, 101
anxiety scale 95
Appleby Report 18
apps 35
assessment
   of dual diagnosis 135, 136–7
   using CBT 26–9
attention deficit hyperactivity disorder (ADHD) 76, 133
attitudes to dual diagnosis patients 128, 142
auditory hallucinations 136
autonomic hypersensitivity 11
avoidance 96

B

Bandura, A. 24
baseline diary 85
Beck, A. 16, 23
bed, leaving 104
behavioural activation (BA) 84–8
behaviours 26–7
   five areas model 29–30, 85, 87, 88, 92
   problem–solving orientation 97–8
   that challenge 10
Bell, A.C. 97
Bennett–Levy, J. 83
bibliotherapy 16, 17
biological markers 115
biological vulnerability factors 11
bipolar disorder 112
body scan, mindful 77–8
bone health 114
borderline personality disorder (BPD) 39, 65
breathing, mindful 77
British Association of Behavioural and Cognitive
   Psychotherapists (BABCP) 24

bubbles, blowing 78–9
Buddhism 67
bulimia nervosa 112

C

caffeine 132–3, 143
cancer 109–10, 114
cannabis 132, 137, 140
   legalisation of 132
cardiovascular disease 109–10, 113
care, compassion and communication cluster 4–5,
   38–9, 64, 82
care co-ordination 8–9
chain analysis 57–8
chaining 119–20
Change 4 Life campaign 109
change theory (CM) 135, 138, 139–40
children
   mindfulness 76
   recommended levels of physical activity 116
chronic pain 76
circadian rhythm 103
clinical supervision 9
clocks, moving 103
clothing for physical activity 118–19
coaching by telephone 54–5
Coalition government policy 19–20
cocaine 133, 143
cognitive behavioural family interventions 16
cognitive behavioural therapy (CBT) 1, 9, 16,
   22–36, 82
   assessment and formulation 26–9
   behavioural principles 25–6
   cognitive principles 25
   evolution of 23–4
   low intensity *see* low intensity CBT interventions
   role of the mental health nurse 24–5
   sessions 32–5
   triggers and consequences 29–30
   understanding the assessment 30–2
cognitive processing 25
cognitive restructuring 88–92
collaborative stance 27
collaborative working 141–2
communication, care and compassion cluster 4–5,
   38–9, 64, 82
communication and interpersonal skills 4, 37–8,
   63, 81
computer-assisted therapy 16, 18
confidence 132
   nurse's 141–2

consequences 29–30
contracts 41–2
coping 12
costs of treatment 109–10
crack cocaine 143
Crawford, M.D. 113
'critical point' 12

D
Dawson, M.E. 10
'DEAR MAN' skills 53
Department of Health (DH) 113, 114–15,
    117, 121
    Dual Diagnosis Good Practice Guide 127, 129
    recommendations for physical activity 115–16
depressant drugs 143
depression 5, 14–15, 83, 84, 101, 134
    mindfulness 75
    physical activity 111–12
describing 68, 72
diabetes 109–10, 113–14
diagnostic overshadowing 128
Diagnostic Statistical Manual (DSM) criteria 31
dialectical behavioural therapy (DBT) 2, 9, 16, 17,
    37–62
    distress tolerance 44–7
    effectiveness 40–1
    emotional regulation 49–52
    history 39
    interpersonal effectiveness 52–5
    mindfulness 47–8, 66
    role of nurses and other professionals 59–60
    sessions 56–8
    skills modules 44–55
    skills training 43–4
    stages of treatment 41–3
diaries
    baseline 85
    behavioural activation 86–7
    cognitive restructuring 89–92
    mood ratings and physical activity 121
    sleep 102
    training schedules/diaries 118
diary card 56–7
diazepam 143
distal vulnerability factors 11
distraction techniques 94, 96
distress 12, 90
    SUDS 94, 95
distress tolerance 44–7
dopamine 133
dual diagnosis 2, 125–46
    clinical approaches 135, 138
    defining 127–8
    intervening in 135–42
    nursing and 127
    nursing assessment and interventions 135,
        136–7
    presentation 129–35
Dual Diagnosis Good Practice Guide 127, 129
Dunkley, C. 54
D'Zurilla, T.J. 97

E
eating disorders 76, 112, 123
ecstasy 144
education
    sleep hygiene 102–3
    psycho-education 93, 135, 138, 139–40
effectively mindful 68, 74
Ellis, A. 23
emotion mind 47, 48, 61
emotion wheel 89, 90
emotional experiences 50–2
emotional regulation 49–52
emotions 26–7, 89–90
    five areas model 29–30, 85, 87, 88, 92
    observing 71–2
    warranted and unwarranted 51
environment, and sleep problems 103
Epictetus 23
Equity and Excellence: Liberating the NHS 19
Essential Skills Clusters 2–3, 4–5, 23, 38–9, 64, 82, 108,
    125–6
everyday mindfulness 70–1
exercise *see* physical activity
exposure chart 96, 97
exposure planning sheet 95
exposure tasks 95
exposure therapy 92–7
    barriers to success 95–7
external stressors 10

F
'FAST' skills 54
Feigenbaum, J.D. 41
field-specific standards 3
fight/flight response 93
five areas model 29–30, 85, 87, 88, 92
football groups 117
formulation 26–9
*From Values to Action: The Chief Nursing Officer's review of
    mental health nursing* 20
fun, physical activity and 118
functionality 83–4

G
garden projects 117
Garland, A. 88
Generalised Anxiety Disorder assessment (GAD 7) 31–2
generic standards 3
genetic vulnerability factors 11
Get Self Help website 28
'GIVE' skills 54
goal setting 86
    physical activity 118
government recommendations for physical activity
    115–16
graded exposure 92–3, 95
    rules of graded exposure therapy 93–4
graded principle 93–4, 96

H
habituation 93
harm minimisation (HM) 135, 140

harm reduction (HR) 138, 139, 140, 141
Heard, H.L. 56
herbal highs 133
heroin 143
hierarchy of competing motivations 119
high energy drinks 143
homeostasis 110
homework 33–4
'hot cross bun' model 27–8, 29–30
'hot thought' 90

I
IAPT (Increasing Access to Psychological Therapies) 18–19, 30, 35, 82
idiosyncratic measures 32
implementation of solutions 100
'IMPROVE' technique 45
in vivo exposure 93
information gathering 26–7
insight into problems 98
interagency working 6, 141–2
internal stressors 10
interpersonal communication skills 135, 139–40
    see also communication and interpersonal skills
interpersonal effectiveness 52–5
intoxication, effects in 131, 143–4

J
joint health 114–15

K
Kabat-Zinn, J. 66–7
Kennerly, H. 102–4
ketamine 144
khat 133, 143
King's Fund 20
Kirk, J. 102–4
Kweskin, S. 132

L
Labour government ten-year programme on mental health reform 18
Lazarus, R.S. 24
leadership, management and team working 22
leaving bed 104
legalisation of cannabis 132
levels of physical activity 115–17
lifestyle 104
Linehan, M. 39, 40, 56, 66, 67, 68
    'how' skills 68, 72–4
    'what' skills 68, 69–72
listing solutions 99
Little, S.E. 54
London School of Economics (LSE) 19
low intensity CBT interventions 2, 81–106
    behavioural activation 84–8
    cognitive restructuring 88–92
    exposure therapy 92–7
    and mental health nursing 83–4
    problem-solving therapy 97–100
    sleep hygiene 101–4
    and their evolution 82–3
LSD 144

M
magic mushrooms 144
Making Mental Health Services more effective and accessible 19
mastery 49
medication 8
memory 131, 133
Mental Health Ten Years On: Progress on Mental Health Care Reform (Appleby Report) 18
mephedrone 133
methamphetamine 133, 143
METs (metabolic equivalents of tasks) 116
mindful body scan 77–8
mindful breathing 77
mindfulness 2, 16–17, 63–80
    in children 76
    DBT 47–8, 66
    defining 66–7
    difference from relaxation 67
    everyday mindfulness 70–1
    exercises 77–9
    'how' skills 68, 72–4
    origins 67
    and physical activity 121
    practising 67–70
    time to give to 74–5
    usefulness to nurses 75–6
    wandering mind 74
    'what' skills 68, 69–72
mindfulness-based cognitive therapy (MBCT) 16–17, 75
mood disorders 132–3
Morris, J.N. 113
motivation 119–20
motivational interviewing (MI) 135, 138, 139
multi-media 35
musculoskeletal health 109–10, 114–15
mushrooms, magic 144

N
napping 103
National Institute for Health and Care Excellence (NICE) 18, 75, 82
    Guidelines 6, 18, 101
necessary activities 85–6
needs/wants 53
negative automatic thoughts (NATs) 25
    cognitive restructuring 88–92
    overcoming and physical activity 120–2
    recognising in mental health disorders 89
negative problem-solving orientation 97–8
No Health Without Mental Health 19
non-judgemental mindfulness 68, 69, 72–3
Nuechterlain, K. 10
Nursing and Midwifery Council (NMC)
    code of conduct 109, 127
    Essential Skills Clusters 2–3, 4–5, 23, 38–9, 64, 82, 108, 125–6
    Standards for Pre-registration Nursing Education 2–3, 4, 22, 37–8, 63, 81, 107, 125
nursing practice and decision-making 22, 81, 107

O

observing 68, 69–72
  an object 69–70
  thoughts and emotions 71–2
obsessive-compulsive disorder (OCD) 110–11,
    132, 134
older adults 116
one-mindful mindfulness 68, 74
opiates 134, 143
ordering activities 86
organisational aspects of care 23, 82, 108
outcome behaviour 10
outcome measures 30–2

P

pain, chronic 76
panic disorder 110
paranoia 136–7
participating 68, 72
Patient Health Questionnaire (PHQ 9) 31–2
Penman, D. 64, 65
person-based cognitive therapy (PBCT) 17
personal development plan (PDP) 3
pharmacological treatment 8
physical activity 2, 104, 107–24
  attending to negative thoughts 120–2
  barriers to 117, 118–20
  benefits of 109–15
  cautions 122–3
  cognitive interventions 117–18
  importance of fitness in mental health nursing 109
  recommended levels of activity 115–17
physical health 109–10
  benefits of physical activity 113–15
physical sensations 26–7
  five areas model 29–30, 85, 87, 88, 92
planning activities 86–7
'PLEASE' technique 49
pleasurable activities 85–6
portfolio 3
positive cycles of thought 121, 122
positive experiences, building 49
positive problem-solving orientation 97–8
post-traumatic stress disorder (PTSD) 75–6, 111, 134
prescription cannabis 132
problem list 98
problem-solving orientation 97–8
problem-solving therapy 97–100
  steps of 98–100
professional values 4, 37, 63, 81, 107, 125
pros and cons
  DBT 45–6, 60–1
  problem-solving therapy 99–100
proximal vulnerability factors 11
psychedelic drugs 144
psychodynamic counselling 16, 17
psycho-education (PE) 93, 135, 138, 139–40
psychological make-up 13
psychological vulnerability factors 11
psychosis 11, 113
  mindfulness 76

psychosocial dimension 7–8
psychosocial interventions (PSIs) 1, 4–21
  Coalition government policy 19–20
  defining 5–6
  descriptions 16–18
  IAPT and the Stepped Model of Care 18–19
  Labour government ten-year programme 18
  mental health nursing and 8–9
  theoretical underpinnings 9–15
  types of 15–16

R

radical acceptance 46
ratings of perceived exertion (RPE) 116
reasonable mind 47, 48, 61
recommended levels of physical activity
    115–17
Recovery Approach 20
Red Bull 143
reflection 3, 34
relationships, maintaining 54
relaxation 67
repetition 94, 96
review of outcome 100
reviewing solutions 99–100
revised thoughts 91, 120
routine activities 85–6

S

schizophrenia 132
sedentary behaviour 116, 121
self-harm 54–5, 136
self-medication hypothesis 131
self-respect, maintaining 54
self-soothe box 44, 60
self-soothing 44–5, 137
situation (trigger) 29–30, 85, 87, 88, 89–90, 92
skills modules 44–55
skills training 43–4
sleep diary 102
sleep hygiene 101–4
sleep problems 101
SMART goals 118
smoking cessation 112–13
social phobia 111
solutions 99–100
solvents 144
Spring, B. 9–10
staged/stepped approach 135
Standards for Pre-registration Nursing Education 2–3,
    4, 22, 37–8, 63, 81, 107, 125
Start active, stay active 109
states of mind in DBT 47–8
Stepped Model of Care 18–19
stimulants 132–3, 143
stress-vulnerability model 9–15
  defining stress 10–11
  defining vulnerability 11
  importance to mental health 14–15
  using psychosocial interventions informed
    by 13–14

stressors 10, 13
subjective measures 32
substance abuse 75
   common features with mental health problems
      129, 130
   dual diagnosis *see* dual diagnosis
   physical activity 112
SUDS (subjective units of distress) 94, 95
suicide 54–5, 136
supervision, clinical 9
support groups 16, 17
Swales, M.A. 56

T
'talk test' 116
team working 55–6
technology
   computer-assisted therapy 16, 18
   and delivering CBT 34–5
   stimuli and sleeping problems 103
telephone coaching 54–5
termination of treatment 42–3
therapeutic relationship
   DBT 56
   dual diagnosis 129–30
third-wave cognitive therapies 16–17
thought diary 89–92
thoughts 26–7
   five areas model 29–30, 85, 87, 88, 92
   hot 90
   observing 71–2
   problem-solving orientation 97–8
   revised 91, 120
time
   dual diagnosis and treatment outcomes 138
   and physical activity 118
   for practising mindfulness 74–5

time *cont.*
   principle in exposure therapy 94, 96
   sleep advice 103
training 9
   skills training in DBT 43–4
training schedules/diaries 118
transtheoretical change models 135, 138, 139–40
treatment pessimism 128, 135
triggers (situations) 29–30, 85, 87, 88, 89–90, 92
type 2 diabetes 109–10, 113–14

U
unwarranted emotions 51

V
validated measures 30–2
values, professional 4, 37, 63, 81, 107, 125
vocational support 16, 18
Volkswagen 121
vulnerability
   defining 11
   stress-vulnerability model 9–15

W
walking 117
wandering of the mind 74
wants/needs 53
Warburton, D.E.R. 113
warranted emotions 51
Westbrook, D. 28, 102–4
Williams, C. 29, 88
Williams, M. 64, 65
willingness 46
wise mind 44, 47–8, 61
withdrawal effects 131, 143–4
   alcohol 132, 145
World Health Organisation (WHO) 109, 115, 128